THE UNOFFICIAL GUIDE TO

SURVIVING PREGNANCY

WITHOUT LOSING YOUR MIND

Edited by

Tiffany O'Connor & Lyndee Brown

ISBN: 0692143858
ISBN-13: 978-0692143858 (HCCR Books)

THIS BOOK IS DEDICATED TO THE PEOPLE WHO
DELIVERED OUR BABIES. THE OB/GYN DOCTORS,
RESIDENTS, NURSES, MIDWIVES, & GAIL'S HUSBAND.
THE CONTRIBUTORS IN THIS BOOK THANK YOU
FOR HELPING US SAFELY BRING OUR
CHILDREN INTO THE WORLD!

SPECIAL THANK YOU TO DIANA LEMUS AND JAMES
O'CONNOR FOR SHARING YOUR QUOTES IN THIS BOOK.

CONTENTS

Foreword.. ix

Section 1: After The Positive Test...................................... 1

1. Congratulations! Now What? 3
2. Pregnancy Announcement: Be Careful Who You Tell!.................... 7
3. The Framed Ultrasound 9
4. Strollers, and Finger Nail Clippers, and Scanner Guns, Oh My!... 14
5. Act like The Pregnant Queen That You Are 18

Section 2: Crash Course in Pregnancy 21

6. What to Really Expect When You Are Expecting...................... 23
7. The Truth about Pregnancy.. 26
8. Pregnancy is Hard and Miraculous................................ 31

Section 3: Pregnancy Symptoms 101 35

9. Pregnancy Symptoms That You Will Love!.................................. 37
10. Pregnancy Symptoms That You Will Hate!.................................. 41
11. Pregnancy Symptoms That Might Scare You! 46

Section 4: Pregnancy Story Time 51

12. During Pregnancy, Puke Happens. Take Advice With a Grain of Saltine.. 53
13. During Pregnancy, Crap Happens. It Helps to Have a Sense of Humor. 56
14. The Itchy Pregnancy.. 60
15. Pregnancy is All the Rage 64
16. I Thought I Knew.. 68
17. It's OK to Dislike Being Pregnant 73
18. My So-Called Average Pregnancy................................ 77

19. My Sweet Surrogacy Journey 82

20. Worth the Wait: The Joy of a Rainbow Baby 87

21. When All You Can Do is Hope, Pray, and Wait 92

Section 5: Your Growing Family **97**

22. All You Need Is Optimism and Hot Dogs 99

23. First Comes Love Then Comes Baby 103

24. How Strange: The Second Baby is Different than the First 109

25. Gender Disappointment: Bonding With Baby the Second
    Time Around 113

26. Tickled Pink 117

Section 6: Tales From The Labor Room **121**

27. How Preterm Labor Changed My Life............................. 123

28. My Last Pregnancy: An Induction Story.......................... 127

29. Vaginal Birth: Advice from Aunt Patti the Great. 130

30. Lifestyles of a Woman in Labor…
    C-section Wishes and Percocet Dreams 135

31. Pregnancy is Unpredictable... 138

32. My Thirty Minute Emergency At Home Labor 143

Section 7: Beyond Pregnancy **149**

33. Breastfeeding: Five Things Your Lactation Consultant
    Failed to Mention 151

34. The Botched Epidural from Hell 154

35. Joy Reclaimed - How Postpartum Depression Refined Me,
    but Didn't Define Me 158

36. What I Wish I Knew When I Was Pregnant About
    Becoming a Mother 163

37. Eating Chocolate in the Bathroom: Tips on Motherhood 168

About the Authors..173

Letter from the Editor...183

FOREWORD

I've had two babies in my life (as far as I know) and both times it was a whirlwind of emotion, anxiety, joy and sheer terror.

Was that normal? Should I be this scared? I feel like I should be more prepared. How the hell have women done this for gabillions of years?! Who ate my last cookie?!

This book is like a group of great friends sharing stories and insights that tell it like it is without scaring the shit out of you. You know the kind of friends I mean, the ones who lean over and give you the brutal truth about weird hair growth but you somehow come away feeling better. They will make you laugh, maybe cry, and hopefully feel less alone while making this person (or people) from scratch. This book is full of great tips and truths, and I wish it had been around when I was pregnant.

Even though pregnancy and new motherhood can sometimes feel scary, gross, exhausting and dropkick frustrating, it truly is an amazing thing that you're doing. You're now part of a club that has walked this crazy path too, so welcome to the tribe and enjoy the ride!

You've got this, kid.

Amy Morrison

Founder of Pregnant Chicken

After The Positive Test

CONGRATULATIONS! NOW WHAT?

MARY ANN BLAIR

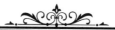

> *"Invest in some comfy flip-flops. By the end of the third trimester, they will be your go-to pair of shoes. Either because none of your shoes fit anymore, or because tying shoes will feel like an Olympic event."*
> *- Miracles in the Mess*

Congratulations, mama! With that positive test, you have officially begun the new adventures of pregnancy and motherhood. Welcome to the club! When I found out I was pregnant, the stick had barely dried before I was at a local bookstore, sifting through the selection of pregnancy books. I couldn't wait to find out what the next nine months had in store for me. While these books were packed with a wealth of medical information, they sorely lacked in practical pregnancy advice…the kind you would want from a girlfriend who has been there, done that and isn't afraid to tell it like it is. I hope that what I'm about to share will serve you well as your tiny embryo grows into your little bundle of joy.

First things first. Find a doctor you genuinely like.

I recommend taking this step as early as possible. While you can't guarantee he/she will be available when your baby enters the world, you will be going to many (and I mean many) appointments over the next nine months. Trust me when I say, you will want to like this person! Find someone you can ask the embarrassing questions to. Someone that will make you feel as comfortable as possible as they poke their fingers into your cervix during those lovely dilation checks. Someone who will give you a sympathetic look as you plead for an epidural or glare at them through a contraction. I know it can be a pain to switch, but your doctor can play a significant role in your overall pregnancy experience. It is worth finding someone you connect with.

On a side note: Expect your doctor to be running way behind schedule from time to time. This used to annoy me. Then one day in my pregnancy brain haze, it dawned on me that my doctor was running late because he had been out delivering a baby. Yeah, it took me awhile to connect the dots. Bring a good book to your appointment (like this one, perhaps?) and enjoy an excuse to sit down and read for forty-five minutes!

Check modesty at the door.

For reals. There are parts of pregnancy that you will wish you didn't know about ahead of time. Group B Strep test, anyone? If you don't know what I'm talking about, feel free to google it. Or don't, because then you might want to skip your next appointment. Of course, the day I had this test done, my doctor was being shadowed by a young, good-looking medical student who needed practice with this procedure. I wished for a stunt double that day! I guess it was a good warm-up for labor and delivery, where I knew I would have to lay it all out there. For my fellow shy gals, I have good news for you! When you are in the midst of labor, you really won't care about who sees what. My first son had a complicated delivery, so by the time he arrived, I had a whole roomful of people with a front row seat to my lady parts. By that point, the entire cast of Grey's Anatomy could have been in the room, and it wouldn't have even phased me! I just wanted him OUT! After delivery, one or both of your boobs will probably be on display as you try to get the baby to latch. Medical professionals have seen it all, so don't give it a second thought.

It is entirely ok if you don't love pregnancy.

With my first son, I was so sick the first trimester that I lost twelve pounds. It was the worst diet I have ever been on. I was throwing up from sunup to sundown. I tried EVERYTHING, and nothing helped. There were times that the only pregnancy glow I had was just the grease in my hair from not having showered for days on end because being upright for any length of time was too much to handle. Finally, around week sixteen, I started to feel better. With my second son, there were fewer hours spent hugging the toilet, but nausea stuck around the ENTIRE nine months. Did I mention the hemorrhoids, varicose veins, swollen ankles, and constipation? Those were a real treat as well. Don't get me wrong, I loved the ultrasounds and feeling my babies kick and grow inside my belly was pretty spectacular. But overall, did I enjoy pregnancy? That would be a big fat NO. Ladies, if you are having one of those pregnancies where you are miserable and counting down the days to your due date, I completely get it. If you are one of the lucky ones with zero morning sickness, a beautiful glowing complexion, and svelte ankles, I have no idea what that is like, but it sounds amazing!

Trust your instincts

When I was around thirty-four weeks pregnant with my first baby, I started having horrendous back pain and felt like I had to pee constantly. When these issues persisted after a couple of days, I called the on-call doctor at the hospital. He explained these symptoms were just the joys of the third trimester and told me to suck it up. (Yeah, he wasn't the nicest.) I had never been pregnant before, and I knew peeing a bunch and back pain was all a part of the gig, so I tried to just soldier on. Then it continued to get worse, so I decided to get checked out to be sure I wasn't in the early stages of labor. It turns out I had a bladder infection and a kidney stone. The moral of the story? Trust your gut. If things don't feel right, don't be afraid to ask questions!

Despite what your relatives say, you have no legal obligation to tell them the baby's name or gender.

We kept the chosen name secret with both our boys. It drove some family members crazy, and they would hound us about the name. As you can imagine, this only made my resolve stronger. I will admit that in a moment of pure relaxation, I told my massage therapist the name we had chosen for our first son. Her reaction was less than awesome. I decided then and there that I would not tell another soul the rest of the pregnancy. My husband and I loved the name, and that is what was important. My rule of thumb? If you played a role in making the baby, you get to have an opinion. Otherwise? Zip it. If you want to keep the name a secret, don't let anyone guilt you into telling! If you're going to keep the gender a secret, more power to you! If you want to tell everyone you know? Go for it! It's your baby, and you get to choose what you do with this information!

Take pictures of your belly.

Toward the end of my pregnancy, when I felt like the Goodyear blimp, I honestly didn't want to take any pictures of myself. My ankles were swollen, my chin had tripled, I could barely squeeze into any of my maternity clothes, but I faithfully took a picture every week to document my expanding midsection, and now I'm so glad I did. I can look at these pictures and embrace my body for what it was…a badass baby growing machine. I highly encourage you to capture these moments. Appreciate your body in all its swollen glory. It's doing a fantastic thing!

One of the scariest parts of pregnancy for me was knowing that, eventually, the baby was going to have to come out somehow! This thought was both exhilarating and terrifying. **Spoiler alert:** Eventually, your baby will have to come out too. In the meantime, I hope you are enjoying the unique experiences pregnancy brings as you await the arrival of your little person. You are about to experience a love you have never known. Once again, **congratulations, mama!**

PREGNANCY ANNOUNCEMENT: BE CAREFUL WHO YOU TELL!

SUNAYNA PAL

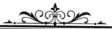

> *"Expect the unexpected. You have no idea what you are capable of. Trust your instincts and yourself."*
> *- Sunayna Pal*

My husband and I moved to a small town in Connecticut from India. This was our fifth move after marriage, and since we were going to stay here for over a year, we decided to try for a baby. My husband was with me when I took the home pregnancy test. The first thing I did after seeing the two pink lines was...well I cried, but the next thing I did was call my mom and tell her about our good news.

She was happy, but like every other mother, she had a list of warnings and tips to give me.

The first instruction she gave me was:

"Do not tell anyone and don't put it on Facebook or any WhatsApp group."

I found that advice odd as I wasn't planning to do anything of that sort, so I just said "OK."

"I mean it."

"Ok, mom. I don't plan to tell anyone via Facebook."

"Don't share it on WhatsApp like you did that time you told everyone about your sister's promotion."

"I won't."

"Good."

With this, she told me not to lift anything heavy and to take care of myself. She continued to give me the standard set of instructions that every pregnant woman gets to hear from every mother she meets. The call went on for about fifteen minutes, and she ended with the same warning she had given me before.

"Don't put it on Facebook!"

I told her that I wouldn't, and my husband and I got on with our day. We decided to follow my mother's advice and not tell anyone. It was slightly difficult because I wanted to tell the whole world, but we kept our lips sealed.

And then I got a text from my aunt, "Good morning Sunu." I hadn't heard from her since we moved to the United States and I found it very odd that she was texting me out of the blue. I returned her greetings, and her next comment confirmed my suspicions that my mother didn't keep her lips sealed.

"I hope that you are taking good care of yourself."

A few hours later, my mom's sister, who also lives in the United States, called me and asked me how I was doing. It didn't take me very long to figure out that she knew about my good news and I knew who had told her.

Eventually, the inevitable happened. One of my aunts who is pretty active on Facebook let me know that she was pleased to hear the good news.

There was no stopping it now. By the next day, everyone knew.

To cut a long story short, if you want to keep your good news a secret, don't tell your mother about it. If there is something that could make a woman happier than knowing she is going to be a mother it is finding out that is she is going to be a grandmother.

THE FRAMED ULTRASOUND

MICHELLE PRICE

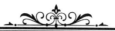

> *"Remember that motherhood is not a competition. There's nothing guaranteed to make you more unhappy or stressed than comparing your pregnancy to someone else's or worrying that your child didn't roll over as fast as another child."*
> *- Honest & Truly*

In the days before Pinterest was a thing, we had to get creative all on our own. Sometimes it worked well - like the baseball cupcakes I made for my son's first birthday that actually looked like baseballs. Other times things didn't go as planned-like when I decided to find a creative way to tell my mom that I was pregnant. I guess it just goes to show that if something wonky is going to happen, it is going to happen in my family.

My husband and I discovered I was pregnant at the beginning of December. We quickly realized that a Christmas reveal, when we're with all our family, was the perfect fit.

Who knew a simple idea could go so wrong?

Without tons of websites to scour, I came up with my own creative idea. I'm positive no one ever thought of this before me. Eh, who am I kidding? My crafting and creativity genes only go so far.

Regardless, I decided to frame our first ultrasound and wrap one up for my parents and one for my husband's parents. What could be a better Christmas present? I briefly debated placing the framed photo in a box with artistically arranged diapers, but artistic arranging isn't my strong suit.

I carefully cut the ultrasound images to create an even border of white on all sides and measured. Being left-handed, this alone presented a challenge. My mom always joked that my only bad grade came in kindergarten when we learned to cut with scissors. No surprise, I ended up with a much smaller border around the ultrasound than I'd initially intended.

Once I finished my cutting masterpiece, I had the easy part. Slap that sucker into a frame and call it a day. My first attempt involved a frame I had on hand in our house.

Of course, as desperately as I tried an ultrasound doesn't fit a standard frame. My pregnancy hormones had me attempting the impossible task for far longer than I should have. In frustration - possibly days later - I finally gave up and carefully shopped for a new frame.

I finally found the perfect frame that wouldn't suggest a gender we neither could know at the time nor would know before my daughter entered the world. I already knew I couldn't deal with another seven months of families trying to tear apart every statement I made or outfit I chose to wear in a vain attempt to be the first to know whether we would have a boy or a girl.

I carefully placed the ultrasound into a gorgeous wood frame with a gender-neutral green matting. Matting - for the non-crafty among us - is a godsend when it comes to making any photos look artistic and pretty. Suddenly, you're Picasso!

The frame went into a flat rectangular box that I carefully wrapped with festive Christmas paper in anticipation of the day. It was so hard not to give it to my mom early or to spill the beans, but I resisted, excitedly waiting for the big reveal.

On Christmas morning, my husband, one-year-old son, and I headed to my parents' house to celebrate.

Once we enjoyed lunch, we started opening presents. As my mom gazed in adoration at her only grandchild, she started waxing poetic. "He's the best baby ever. You have the perfect family. It's so nice with him, especially now that he's developing such a fun personality."

I smiled, knowing we had a secret but not wanting to spoil the surprise. My mom loved my son so much so of course, she'd love a second child - especially since my sister and I were only 15 months apart. She knew and enjoyed kids close in age.

Finally, she opened her presents. I kept a careful eye on her every movement to ensure I didn't miss a second of her grandma excitement. When she got to the flat rectangular one, I set aside everything I had in my hands and watched her with expectant glee.

She carefully unwrapped it and stared down at the image in front of her.

I clasped my hands, trying not to bounce out of my seat with excitement. I couldn't wait to hear my mom's reaction and patiently - ok, not so patiently - waited for her to speak.

Eventually, she looked up with a blank expression. "Why are you giving me a picture of an owl?"

An owl? Wait, what? An owl? Hold on...SHE'S SERIOUS.

"Uhhhhhh, Mom, that isn't an owl. Look again."

She peered at the ultrasound carefully once more. "Is that Farrell?" "No, Mom. I didn't give you a picture of my cat either."

Although I kept my happy facade in place, I felt my heart begin to sink. She didn't recognize the ultrasound. As I thought back to my first pregnancy, I realized I might not have shared an ultrasound with her, as she'd lived two states away until four days after my son was born.

Maybe she'd never seen an ultrasound before? But hasn't everyone? Doesn't she watch t.v? Can't she see inside my mind and just know?

"Look closely at the sides. Do you see the writing?"

She picked up her reading glasses - and that should have been my first clue, aside from the fact that my son was her only grandchild. As she looked more closely, her puzzled look slowly cleared.

She smiled at me. "I have no idea what this is."

I blinked at her in utter incomprehension. My jaw hit the floor, and I may have let out a small sob. Did she not know the hours I put in creating the perfect borders around that ultrasound? The useless attempts to fit it into a frame that almost resulted in me ripping up the ultrasound in frustration? The way I selected the perfectly artistic matting to put in the pretty frame that would set off the baby in the middle of it?

My perfectly planned oh-so-clever reveal was not going as planned. That's when the pregnancy hormones took over again, and I blurted out that I was pregnant. Couldn't she see that was my ultrasound? I sniffled through my explanation, waiting for her to jump up from her seat in the excitement I'd felt just moments before.

My mom sat back in her chair. "So all this time I was talking about your perfect family and how you couldn't possibly make life better... all the comments I made today about you not needing or wanting another baby... that might not have been exactly in the best taste, huh?"

I nodded tearfully, and she finally gave me the hug I so desperately needed. "I'm sure we'll find the room in our hearts for another baby. But after two - you are done, right? I don't think I can handle having a third child." The last statement came with the eyebrow raise all mom's perfect within an hour of giving birth.

I meekly nodded. Fortunately, my husband and I had only ever planned on having two children.

Our announcement may not have gone quite the way we planned with my mom, but my mother in law took one look at her own beautifully framed ultrasound and knew exactly what it was. Thank goodness!

If you're currently pregnant, be grateful you have the world of Pinterest at your fingertips to identify the best way to announce to your - potentially clueless - family that you're about to bring a bundle of joy into the world. A framed ultrasound? That may or may not be the way to go.

After all, you wouldn't want your mom thinking you planned to birth an owl.

STROLLERS, AND FINGER NAIL CLIPPERS, AND SCANNER GUNS, OH MY!

AMY WEATHERLY

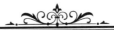

> *"If you are holding this book right now, breathe. Chances are you are going to be an amazing mother. Not because this book holds any magical secrets, but because you are already the kind of mom who wants and pursues and searches for what's best for her children."*
> *- Amy Weatherly, Writer*

Everything about my pregnancy was a total surprise. I mean...I guess it really shouldn't have been. I was twenty-seven years old and married, and we were too broke to afford cable, so we were doing lots of, you know, "it."

Looking back, we really shouldn't have been so shocked. If preventatives only work ninety-nine times out of one hundred, then it all makes sense.

But there we were: pregnant, broke and beyond terrified.

I had only changed one diaper in my life. One. And the last time I babysat, one of the little girls fell off of the swing and hit her head on the ground and another one bit through a teething ring, and I spent all night searching the Internet for a list of the ingredients inside teething rings. (Water. They're filled with water, but I was so ignorant that I honestly had no clue.) And another one was able to talk me out of going to bed on time.

I got bamboozled by a five-year-old. Nothing about my college degree prepared me for kids.

So saying I felt unqualified to be a mother was the understatement of the year. Fun - yes. Smart - depends on which former teacher you ask.

Nice - most of the time, but don't cut me off on the highway. Mother material - yeah, that's going to be a hard pass. I didn't have it.

So I'm chugging along through my pregnancy - reading everything, Googling everything, asking my doctor about everything, doubting everything, eating ev-er-y-thing - and it comes time to register. That's fun, right? That's a good time.

I'm not super shallow, but I am regular shallow, and I love me some gifts. And gifts that I've specifically asked for: wheeeee howdy, well everyone knows, those are the best kind.

So I walk into Babies 'R Us (May she Rest in Peace), hand in my hubby's, massive smile on my face. We fill out the paperwork, and they hand me the gun. Ohhhhhh the scanner gun. I just felt better with it in my hand. I felt like my entire life had been leading up to this exact moment.

First thing: stroller.

Ummmmmm...

"Ma'am, can you tell me the difference between these? Why is this one six hundred dollars and this one sixty dollars? Are the tires different? Is the quality that different? Does a stroller really need to be made out of the same material as my husband's giant truck? Is my baby going to fall out of the cheap one? Will the expensive one change diapers for me? Is it made out of gold? What's the deal here?"

"I don't know. You're just going to have to read the descriptions."

Ok, now I see why maybe things didn't work out for that store. What? Did I just say that? Am I allowed to say that? Whatever...it's true. Customer service, people. And brains. And commissions. You're here to make money, yes? Convince me to get the more expensive one. I'm young and dumb and likely to chomp on that bait.

Ok, anyways.

So right from the start, I felt helpless and completely overwhelmed.

In my immense amount of knowledge and smarts, I thought to myself: "You went too big, too fast. Start small and build your way up."

Good in concept. Bad in theory. There are more options when it comes to small, cheap things. And for a hormonal woman already on the verge of tears, too many choices is a complete and utter nightmare.

So my hubby and I headed to the body care aisle for fingernail clippers.

My word. Have you been down this aisle? There's so much. Why is there so dang much? Why are there so many options from the same brand? Make one. Make one excellent one that encompasses all the best qualities and us consumers will just buy that one. Don't make us choose.

What if I pick the wrong one? What if I don't get the right fingernail clippers and clip his nails too short, and he bleeds to death?

OH MY ACTUAL GOSH. The thoughts began to spiral out of control, and stack themselves one on top of the other.

I have ten of my own fingernails to cut. And now I'm going to have ten more. That's twenty friggin' fingernails to be in charge of! I am not ready for this.

And at that moment, a massive wave of pressure crashed over me, and I literally waddle/ran out of that store in tears. I'm not a teenager or a Kardashian who doesn't know how to use the word correctly. When I say I literally waddle/ran out of that store, I mean that I literally waddle/ran out of the store. Literally. And collapsed into a pile of irrational fears and puddles of tears right outside the sliding glass door.

I'm sure everyone was staring. I'm not dramatic or anything, ever. I don't make a scene, and I definitely don't over-react. Except that I do. Oops...

My husband, who likes to follow the rules and stay inside the lines, came outside and grabbed the scanning gun from my shaking hands, and brought it back inside and apologized to everyone, and then came back outside to console his crazy wife and find out what the heck just happened in there.

"I can't do it. It's just too much. It's a person, like a real person. I'm about to be in control of another person with actual fingernails, and I ate a whole bag of goldfish crackers and a Wendy's frosty for lunch so clearly I'm not equipped to deal. Nobody should put me in charge of anything or anyone ever. Please don't make me do this."

We ended up going home.

I wasn't ready for it.

So when the time was right, I found an amazing website, Diapers.com in case you're wondering, and just registered on there. I made it simple. I just picked the item with the most stars and BOOM. Done-ski.

And guess what? That baby boy came out, and I did what all good mothers do, I ended up just biting his fingernails off and never even touching the clippers until he was older.

I'm a mother of three now, and I am officially in charge of cutting forty fingernails, and I do it all with grace. Or sometimes I forget, and they go to school looking like zombies, which they love because it gives them the chance to dig in there and pick their noses the way that they like. But I always feed them, and I always make sure they know they are loved, so even though I'm not perfect, we're all going to be just fine in this house.

Upon reflection, I do wish I would've done a better job of appreciating the power of the scanner gun though. I'll never have another chance to use that thing again, unless...

Yeah, this is a brilliant idea. I'm doing it.

...unless I throw myself a lavish thirty-five-year-old birthday party and register for all my gifts.

BRB I have to go to Nordstrom's real quick

ACT LIKE THE PREGNANT QUEEN THAT YOU ARE

LYNDEE BROWN

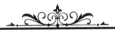

> *"Pregnancy is the only time in your life when people won't question you. You could walk through a room carrying a shovel, rope, and lye and everyone would be like...aww, isn't she cute, she has to be about seven months pregnant."*
> ~ *#Lifewithboys*

The one thing I can tell you about pregnancy is that no one, I mean NO ONE will have the exact same experience as you. However, every mother will want to tell you how her pregnancy went and compare stories. I too am guilty of this need to overshare. Is it annoying at times, especially when it's some random stranger in a grocery store reaching for your belly and taking TWENTY MINUTES to tell you things that do not apply to your pregnancy? Yes!!! However, there are some advantages to being pregnant and having everyone want to shower you with attention. Here are some of the pregnancy perks that you need to make sure you enjoy...By the way, you're welcome in advance.

Perk #1: A Baby Shower Is Like Christmas, Have One or Two

Say yes to all of the showers! It is ok to allow more than one person to plan one for you. You probably have a few groups of friends, like lifelong friends and work friends. Say, each group decides to host a baby shower for you. Well, who are you to say no to such a kind offer? Maybe you have family members that don't get along, and each side of the family wishes to throw their own celebration of the life inside of you in an attempt to outdo each other. Don't protest... just take advantage and enjoy all the free stuff for your little angel! It's like Christmas, but all the presents are for your child, and you don't have to pay for them. Free is good. Free is the best! No matter how many diaper cakes you get, you are still going to pay for all of the rest of your child's stuff until they are legally an adult. Nobody gets together and throws a party because little Jimmy needs braces and braces are expensive...so enjoy the free stuff while it lasts.

Perk #2: VIP Parking

Take this from someone who did not have the new or expecting mothers sign at the grocery store, USE IT! If you have to waddle into the store, then waddle your pregnant booty from a close parking space to the door. Everyone avoids that spot hoping that a pregnant person or new mother will use it so they can feel good about themselves for the day. It's like the car drivers version of giving up their seat on the bus for someone who needs it more. Really if you think about it, you are doing the world a favor. And if you just had the baby, you now know how heavy an infant is in their car seat. So use the new mother's parking spot. You are not the Hulk. There will be plenty of other chances during motherhood for martyrdom...like carrying a sixty-pound sleeping five-year-old across a colossal zoo parking lot uphill the entire way. Enjoy the break now while everyone wants to give it to you.

Perk#3: An Excuse to Get All the Pedicures You Want

The other place you get to waddle into guilt-free is the nail salon. I mean have you ever tried to give yourself a pedicure with a basketball or watermelon blocking your way as you bend towards your toes. Unless you are into some serious yoga, it is probably going to be very uncomfortable. You will have to choose between not being able to breathe while the baby is shoved into your diaphragm or being able to clip your nails and get paint on the nail itself. Breathing wins every time, its science. The foot massage, hot stone, and scrub are only secondary to the whole breathing thing, you know, in case your partner wants to know why you are spending all your time at the nail salon, tell them science made you do it.

Perk #4: There IS No Shame in Your Carb Game

All these years you have been watching your carbs. Saying "NO" to this bad carb and that bad carb. Judging yourself and others for all the carbs all the time. Okay so maybe that was me when I was really jealous of someone eating cake in front of me. What I am saying is that there is no judgment when you are pregnant. You get a free pass to the carb buffet. Your feeling like a giant bowl of pasta with *gasp* Alfredo sauce, then eat it. You are feeling like a special cupcake from your favorite bakery, send someone else to get it because they will think it is cute that you have a craving. Also since you are the official designated driver for the next nine months, you can eat extra carbs because you don't have to worry about all those bad carbs in alcohol. It's called balance.

Perk# 5: It Is Your Special Time with the Baby

The best perk is that this is YOUR special time with the baby. The only time it will be just the two of you. During the next nine months, your child is actually connected to you inside your body. All of the sensations in your belly, when the baby hiccups, rolls and, kicks, they are your moments alone to cherish. Every change and moment of growth are moments that you share together. You and the baby are one.

Remember, whether your pregnancy is easy breezy or you are a sick mess, there is something so wonderfully amazing about growing life inside you that it brings out the light in you and shines it like a beacon to others. Enjoy this time to shine because before you know it that baby is here in the flesh and then in a blink of an eye, they are becoming a toddler and then a teenager. Eventually, you will find yourself oddly reaching for a strangers belly at the store and telling her a twenty-minute story about the special cupcakes you craved when you were pregnant.

Crash Course in Pregnancy

WHAT TO REALLY EXPECT WHEN YOU ARE EXPECTING

JOEY FORTMAN

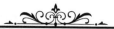

> *"It's ok if you can't breastfeed. Do NOT let anyone else tell you otherwise!! Not all of us are blessed with boobs that milk. You may not be one of the chosen ones, but don't let that kill you. It is OK. It just means that your boobs will stay perkier longer!"*
> *~ Reality Moms*

Motherhood is honestly nothing like I had imagined. I imagined this big, blossomed pomp and circumstance with pixie dust and diapers that magically appear on baby butts. I thought that delivery was a joyful, happy experience that moms celebrated with no pain medicine followed by a glass of champagne at the end. I imagined a hospital room full of flowers and family members who immediately took care of the baby while the new mom got to sleep.

Oh hell. Who on Earth made up motherhood that way? I guess I did. Or the mom on my street who looks like Bree from Desperate Housewives, red hair and all. However, she turned out to be Mary-Louise Parker from Weeds. I have two boys, but fortunately, I don't have to sell marijuana to survive with my men in this world.

When my almost ten-year-old was born, I was a complete and utter disaster. For about three years...yep. This was a mom with just one boy. When the second one came into the picture, God granted me a whole new approach. But let's stick to the insanity, shall we?

Pregnancy: There is this extreme sense of awesomeness that comes along with being pregnant. I was barely a married woman when I got knocked up. (I love that terminology because if you think about it, you ARE knocked up when you are pregnant. The only thing missing is getting 'knocked upside the head'!) When I found out I was pregnant, I expected bells to ring out in celebration and pink and blue candy to fall from the sky. Instead, I found myself face down in the toilet for the first three months. Morning sickness. Constipation. Swollen body parts. Cankles that look like ham hocks. No one tells you about THAT part of motherhood. Make no mistake, no candy falls from the celebration sky. If candy does fall out of the air for you, it probably means that you bugged your hubby enough that he went out, bought it and is now throwing it like confetti over your head. Eat the daylights out of it already!

Eating: Girl, do NOT sit face first at midnight with a gallon of ice cream, go for the pint instead. Do NOT eat an entire pizza just because you think you can...or the bag of Oreos. Gaining weight can cause gestational diabetes, tuna has mercury in it, and cheese...don't even get me started. Avoid that Mexican restaurant you love. No margarita and no Queso dip is HELL, right?

Bathing: I'd say immediately after the first trimester you'll never see your feet again. And if you think you will love showering, you won't. Not when your hair growth down below makes you look like a cavewoman. It is so gross. You would have no idea unless you grew a human in your stomach. Good news though? If you take a bath, you'll float!

Boobs: If you didn't have them before you got pregnant, you very well may not have them during pregnancy or after. In fact, be prepared that they will never look the same. And if you love the way they look? Pfft. Once that human hits Earth there is a big chance your estrogen push after will give you boob hair the length of your middle finger. (Sharing for a friend.)

Brains: If you didn't believe in the excuse called Mom Brain...I can assure you that you'll get it too. There is no hiding or denying this crazy experience. In fact, it makes you feel like a boob when you forget the important things and are consistently called out about it from the overly perfect moms in your neighborhood.

Body: You will see all of these celebrities talking about how quickly they bounced back to their pre-baby selves. Girlfriend, that is FAR from the truth. And those that tell you they do are either lying or a freak of nature. I distinctly remember eating the house and everything in it. I had a large cotton candy flavored ice cream from Dairy Queen like twice a week! Sooo bad...I know. It was the beginning of my demise. Ugh! My baby is ten now. That ice cream weight? STILL THERE.

Bodily Functions: You have no idea. And when you do? I'll be praying for you. Get used to spending time in the bathroom. When you are pregnant, you will have to pee all the time. After pregnancy, you will spend countless hours teaching your child to pee in the toilet. Potty training...It's like dealing with the devil. Ok so maybe not that bad but it sure feels like it sometimes. I remember those days like they were yesterday. Who am I kidding, it was yesterday! Even with a five-year-old and nine-year-old you never have to stop training them to PEE IN THE TOILET! With boys, the amount of pee in your life will give you rage. Especially when it's on your wall, in your carpet, covering your floor...Everywhere but the inside of the toilet! Even on the toilet seat. When I sit in it? Hell hath no fury. My boys run for their lives. I've been known a time or two to wake up the whole house when I go pee in the middle of the night and sit in it.

Are you terrified to become a mom yet? Don't be. There are some amazing moments of motherhood that you'll never forget. Like watching your child successfully hit the potty on a permanent basis or walking your kid to the bus stop for the first time. There is a sense of relief you feel that day, but there will also be a deep sense of sadness. At least there was for me. Sadness because I felt like I missed the first few years of their life focusing on all the silly stressors. Things that didn't matter in the long run.

Whatever you do? Know that you are their chosen one. Whether in the womb or the world, that baby was meant entirely for you. As much as you want to toss a dirty diaper in the face of anyone who tells you they grow up too fast in your parenting heart of hell, step back and agree. This too shall pass.

THE TRUTH ABOUT PREGNANCY

LOUISE SHARP

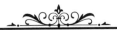

"Through all the sickness and the tiredness, enjoy it. Embrace it. Because one day you'll look back and miss feeling those tiny little flutters which turned into kicks."
- Louise Sharp, Writer

While pregnant with my youngest, I remember my first appointment with the doctor. I remember telling her how about how great I felt, full of energy, and so excited for the months ahead. I was five weeks pregnant.

Let's fast forward to week eight where the pregnancy hormones kicked in. I should have known the drill by now, as this was my third pregnancy. We'd planned it to be our last, and I wanted so badly for it to be different from the others. I wanted to enjoy it more. I wanted to glow. I wanted people to comment how I looked fabulous rather than how big and joking if I was 'sure it's not twins.'

I'm not convinced these perfect pregnancies exist. No matter how much we seem to see them through celebrities in the media or our friends on our social feeds.

I feel that maybe we should talk more honestly and openly about pregnancy and realize it's perfectly okay to admit you're finding it tough, or feeling horrendous and in all honesty, wishing the nine months over, without feeling inadequate, judged or ungrateful.

So, I thought I'd share an insight into what to really expect during pregnancy, based on my own experiences.

'Morning' Sickness

How naive was I when I thought the sickness phase, as commonly described in pregnancy books, would automatically stop at around twelve weeks. Like it's on a timer. For me, it lasted all day, every day, with all three babies. I'm not talking just little bouts of nausea as you go about your day. But a full-on hangover.

I spent the majority of the nine months with my head in the toilet. Any toilet.

I'd say spewing just became part of my morning routine. Wake up, go to the bathroom, and throw up. Maybe it just became some weird habit, who knows.

Baby Brain

The pregnancy-induced fog which many women experience, and scientist 'claim' may exist. It does exist, and we don't need a dude in a white coat in a lab to confirm it.

You'll forget everything where the ability to remember even your own name becomes difficult. I was asked the date of births of my two children while pregnant with my third, along with my due date at a doctor's appointment. All I could offer was a blank stare. For a good few minutes. I ended up skint for four days when I incorrectly entered my pin number in the cash point three times and said goodbye to my card.

It's not just a pregnancy thing either. You'll still be going to Boots for nappies but leaving with toothpaste and finding your keys in the fridge well after the birth. I went for a walk one afternoon not long after having my youngest daughter Emily. I suddenly filled with panic and fear and began to look around as I thought 'Crap, where is Jessica'? Then remembered I'd dropped her off at nursery twenty minutes earlier.

The Sonographer Isn't Always Correct

From my twenty week scan with my first, we eagerly awaited the birth of 'Chloe,' and I built up a collection of pretty little frilly dresses and dinky pink shoes.

Some went back to the shop once Callum arrived into the world at forty-two weeks, and some my sister dressed him in any way for a giggle and photos which we will get blown up for his twenty-first birthday.

Obviously, technology has progressed over the last eighteen years, and they were right on the money with my other two. Still I persuaded my hubby to fork out £120 with both for a private scan to confirm it, though.

I'd suggest holding out on decorating the nursery pink or blue until the little one arrives and have a backup name of the opposite gender. We didn't, but I'd saw Titanic just a couple of months earlier and, really liked the name, Cal. The midwife asked the babies name, and I shouted out 'Callum' while still high on Entonox and pethidine. I'm glad I did.

Sometimes I wonder why I didn't just leave the sex as a surprise, but there is no bigger surprise than expecting a girl but giving birth to a beautiful baby boy.

It's Not Just Nine Months

The first twenty weeks are the longest, although probably not as long as the last two weeks, or the two weeks after your due date. And if you have pregnant friends or know anyone who is due around the same time as you, they'll give birth before you. Guaranteed.

My hubby made the mistake of telling me one of his workmates had just gone on paternity leave as he walked through the door one night. My eyes widened as he realized he shouldn't have done this. She was due after me. I was due pretty much before anyone I knew who dropped before me.

Everything Makes You Cry

News articles, songs, films, pregnancy books, advertisements, the price of prams, everything. Especially the price of prams.

Then there's the other end of the spectrum when you get 'The Rage.' I'm not a jealous partner. And that's not because I'm all confident in myself, I'm not. I don't seem to feel jealousy as an emotion...Except while with child.

My hubby went to an open day at a gym with his friend. I was okay with this at first. Why wouldn't I be? Till I started to envision hot girls in gym gear, with tiny little waists while mine was that of a baby hippo, and then the texts went from 'are you having a good day'?, to 'IS IT ALL MEN' and 'WHEN ARE YOU COMING HOME.' Yeah, I felt a slight niggle of jealousy that day.

The 'Glow'

Spots, dry skin, bloodshot eyes from sickness - absolute radiance.

Food Aversions

I remember smugly discussing diet with my midwife right at the start of my last pregnancy. I had just lost around 50lbs so obviously wanted to gain as least weight as possible, and sat and confidently told her how disciplined I now was and would 100% be sticking to a healthy nutritious diet of fruit and veg.

I could literally only stomach bread, chicken, and mash for around the first five months as I found myself unintentionally on some beige colored food diet as anything with any color made me want to barf.

I gained around 60lbs and only just under 9lb of that was baby, lets attribute about 20lbs to fluid, placenta, boobs, and uterus, and the rest was chocolate, donuts, crisps, biscuits...Fail!

A Heightened Sense of Smell

We're talking that of a bloodhound. It drives you crazy, and it makes you nauseous.

I wasn't living with my now hubby till about seven months into the pregnancy, and he knew to remove all the plug-ins before going to his house. My new sofa got doused in Olbas oil (hubs idea) making the smell even more unbearable than that of leather which was knocking me sick in the first place, and all plastic bags went in the bin. Yes, plastic bags have a smell.

I took the bus home from work during my first pregnancy, and some fool got on with a pizza. I suffered for thirty minutes with the overpowering Meat Feasty smell wafting around in front of me. Ran (waddled quickly) home down the never-ending street (I lived at number 208), knocked frantically on the front door, rushed past my mum and thank goodness there was a downstairs toilet as I made it just in time. Luckily, it doesn't last the whole nine months; I'd say eight.

However, I will be honest, and keep this balanced. It's not all horror stories. The best, most special thing about pregnancy, which you will think about for years and years after giving birth, probably forever, is the tiny little flutters you feel at around sixteen weeks. Which then turn into little patters, then tight squeezed wiggles and kicks which wake you up in the night and keep you awake for hours as you lie and watch growing bump knockout some rather impressive shapes.

It's without a doubt, the best, most precious feeling in the world.

So maybe like almost everything else in your life, the best, most wonderful, most amazing things come from the hardest, darkest and most difficult of times.

PREGNANCY IS HARD AND MIRACULOUS

KAREN SZABO

*"Keep a bottle of Tums by your bed and take
advice with a grain of salt. No one will know
what's going on better than you."*
- The Antsy Butterfly

I heard mixed reviews about pregnancy before I got pregnant. Some women said that it was glorious and painless and an absolute joy while others said it was exhausting and painful and they couldn't wait for it to be over. I didn't know what to expect because, as they say, every pregnancy is different. However, everyone I spoke to agreed that pregnancy – in its entirety – is hard.

Hard? What's so hard about being pregnant? I mean, you're only literally manufacturing a human being inside your own body for roughly 40 weeks. It's not like it's an alien that's going to jump out of our belly and eat your face. We all know what we've signed up for, don't we?

I knew I was pregnant before I took the seven dollar-store pregnancy tests I kept stashed under my bathroom sink for when the time came. The sickness was intense. I ended up having an extended bout of morning – or rather all day – sickness with my pregnancy. Even though I had to take medication throughout my entire pregnancy, I wasn't sure what the big deal was. My being sick was just a minor inconvenience as to what was coming: a baby. A human being. Who cares that there were times when I could be found throwing up in a plastic bag on my lap while on my way home from work? It was all part of this magical experience. Waking up nauseous was just another of the many ways my son was telling me that he was right there, in my uterus, taking up as much energy as he needed from me. Sharing is caring.

And sharing is what I did, the whole time. While my body was busy creating a person, I'd still plug away at the daily duties of life no matter how tired I was. Because things had to be done and being pregnant is no excuse not to do them, even in sheer exhaustion. My boy sucked up my energy like a vacuum, and I let it slide because it was all for the greater good. I pushed aside the heavy eyelids and constant yawns and did what I had to do. I am a team player after all.

As the pregnancy progressed, so did the symptoms. I must have missed the memo about possible painful bowel movements when pregnant because I was in shock the first time it happened. When I realized that I was, in fact, trying to expel a hockey puck from my rear, I got scared. But hey, it's all part of the process, isn't it? No pain no gain, they say. Sure, I had to hold on to the side of the toilet, tears pouring out of my eyes, face as red as a hot pepper, as my husband awkwardly tried to coach me through it. But what's a little constipation in the grand scheme of things? We got to practice our Lamaze breathing techniques, and I got to fit in a bit of reading time while I sat there, waiting, in agony.

Things picked up, though, when sciatica hit. I had no idea what was going on. I thought maybe the baby had pinched one of my nerves. I'd never experienced sciatica, but luckily my husband had. He showed me a few stretches that worked for him, but because my belly was so big, I found his way very difficult. Luckily, I had an excellent pregnancy book by my side, and it offered me a slew of things I could do to diminish the piercing pain I was experiencing, which mostly occurred before bedtime. All it took was a few uncomfortable positions to stretch out that back before being able to go to bed.

Ah, bedtime. What every pregnant woman looks forward to. That time when you can finally relax on one side or the other because we can't lie down on our back due to some massive blood vessel that could potentially cut off the blood supply to our unborn child. But no matter. All it took was a few hours of positioning pillows between my legs and switching sides to avoid getting bed sores. It was a walk in the park! Of course, when the acid reflux kicked in, that complicated matters a bit more. But with the help of a dozen Tums already poured out onto my night-table so that I wouldn't have to wake my husband up with the constant shaking of the bottle, I managed to get a bit of sleep in, and my husband was able to sleep soundlessly throughout the night.

Perhaps the lack of sleep contributes to the emotional vortex we get sucked into while creating life. As someone who lives with depression and anxiety, I may have been a bit more on the moody side. I cried as if I needed to gather enough water to sail a boat to the hospital when the time came to give birth. The hormones scattered like mice when a cat comes into the room and they popped in and out like Jack-In-The-Box without notice and without mercy. Luckily, we have a Costco membership, so we were never low on tissue. It sounds rough, but it's just another signal that everything is going as planned and the baby is doing well. It's a comforting reminder while your head is in the freezer trying to cool yourself down that the end is near, and you'll get to hold the same baby that is currently kicking you in the ribs and spleen.

However, the kicks are kind of cool if you think about it. The baby moves around, and your belly looks like a surfer's paradise the way the waves move in and out. What's a little elbow sticking out of your side as the owner of said elbow stretches out as if they're sleeping on a king-sized bed? I feel bad for the baby, I do. They barely have any room in there. They're all scrunched up and uncomfortable. Of course, they need their stretches. So, when the kicks were hard enough that it felt like a foot was going to bust through my belly button, I remembered what close quarters this poor child was living in and I did my best to shrug it off. I'd put on some peaceful music and rocked my body back and forth, desperately trying to calm the little person living inside of me.

Because pregnancy is all sorts of fun, another symptom that pregnant women endure is water retention. Our feet and hands swell like balloons. Even our faces swell, mine did. It's disappointing when we can no longer fit in our loosest pair of shoes or biggest pair of flip-flops. At least no one is going to die of dehydration.

Of course, after forty weeks of piecing together a human being, all of the above symptoms can become overwhelming. So when the baby refuses to come out and you're already a few days overdue, it's only natural to get a bit frustrated. It's entirely understandable that you may be a bit more snappy than usual or start calling your husband names. But fear not. The baby will come when it is ready to come.

No delivery would be complete without experiencing some form of discomfort or complication, including ones involving an emergency C-section. It may be a frightening time in our lives, but at the end, when it is all over, you get to hear the cries of that tiny human being you spent so much time making. All of the other stuff washes away like water over a smooth rock, and as soon as you're able to stop shaking from the immense amount of drugs they put you on, you get to hold your baby.

Despite what you go through while pregnant, keep in mind that you made a person, and that, in itself, is pretty miraculous.

Pregnancy Symptoms 101

PREGNANCY SYMPTOMS THAT YOU WILL LOVE!

ALISON CHRUN

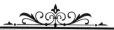

"No matter what anyone tells you, there will be highs, there will be lows, and there will be a beautiful, unique experience you will never forget. Enjoy your pregnancy journey and embrace the changes."
- Appetite for Honesty

I always imagined I would be one of those women who hated being pregnant. Bottom line, I don't love being inconvenienced, so I never thought I'd thrive off of a nine-month alien invasion. More than likely I'd lie helplessly in bed while my minions (ahem, family) waited on me hand and foot in anticipation of 'the end.'

Well, after realizing that if I wanted to procreate, I would have to consider getting pregnant, the joke was on me. As it turned out, I did the whole alien invasion thing pretty damn well. And liked it so much, I did it one more time for shits and giggles.

As much as I'd heard about the aches and pains of carrying another human, I dreaded that whole 'pushing out the human' part. It just seemed painful and truly terrifying. But I accepted my fate and began trying. After some time, I fell pregnant, and I say "fell" because well, I almost fainted. Finding out you're pregnant is the equivalent to being at the peak of the first hill of the tallest roller coaster in the world, and knowing there's no way off the ride except down.

Would my strength as a woman carry me through these next nine months with grace, or should I plan to vacate my real life for the duration of this pregnancy to spare my loved ones the nuisance I'd inevitably become?

I expected to hate pregnancy. I expected never to want to do it again. One and DONE! But what I didn't expect, were all the things I'd LOVE about it.

BOOBS BOOBS BOOBS

I wasn't blessed with much of a chest, but six weeks into my pregnancy and BAM! There they were, full, firm and the perfect size for my frame. Sure the small amounts of leakage over the next seven months were a little annoying, but nothing to complain about in exchange for these beautiful babies! It was the most natural, perfect boob job! And for those who were blessed with a chest and hate this first 'pro" to pregnancy, my condolences. The grass is always greener, right?

Luscious, Thick, Shiny Hair Don't Care

Before becoming pregnant, I read that it wasn't good for the baby to get your hair dyed or highlighted, especially in the first trimester. So, there went my happiness. I used to get my hair done religiously every three months, and it was the only "Me" time I was genuinely committed to until my prenatal pills and hormones kicked in. Not only was my hair growing as rapidly as a Chia Pet, but it was also thick, and shiny! It felt like my hair was on steroids and I couldn't get enough! I got so many compliments on my hair; I convinced myself this was just how my hair would look the rest of my life. And while I mourned the postpartum hair loss as if my favorite pet died, it was worth it for the nine months of hair commercial hair I had. I'll always cherish that time my hair and I had together.

Period-be-GONE

Need I say more? Aside from the natural cramping AKA growing pains of the pregnant belly, not bleeding every Twenty-eight days is AMAZING! As women know, Aunt Flo is one of the most unwelcomed guests of our lifetime, and yes, when she doesn't show up, we FREAK OUT, panic and go to every extreme possible to figure out what is wrong with us, but ultimately we'd still prefer her to never show up at our front door again. The nine months and change that we don't have to see Aunt Flo's face is the most blissful months without her. Yes, she will make her comeback with a vengeance and stick around longer than her usual stay, but those nine months are worth it. I love that the only time I'd know what it was like to be a man, without a period, would also coincide with growing a human. This is why women are warriors.

Guilt-Free Eating Habits

I have to say that with my first pregnancy, I ate ALL THE THINGS! I never had a sweet tooth before pregnancy, but I adopted one in my first pregnancy and never once did I feel guilty about it. I never felt bad about giving into cravings, and made sure everyone knew that I was eating for two; even though scientists say that's not really a thing, but what the hell do they know? I gained the most weight in my first pregnancy, and since then, I called that pregnancy a learning curve. I had to give in, to learn what my body could take, and boy did I learn!

My second pregnancy was an entirely different story. I was determined not to gain as much weight, and therefore, I didn't give in as much to cravings. I was a little more mindful of what I consumed, and when I say "a little," I mean it. I still indulged, and ate for two and ate my weight in chocolate, but I incorporated exercise into that pregnancy, which I never did in my first. I used my first pregnancy as an excuse to sit on my butt and avoid all things involving physical exertion.

So, you CAN have it all. You CAN have the best of both worlds. Just be sure to have two kids and the first go-round, go big or go home. The second go-round, walk the block once a day, and you'll be all good!

Excuses, Excuses

I'm a pretty honest and blunt person. I like to tell it like it is. But in pregnancy, sometimes we don't have the energy to be honest, because then there has to be a detailed explanation and who has time for that? So, when someone asked me to do something or go somewhere that I didn't want to do or go, I'd point to my belly and say, "NOPE," and no one questioned me otherwise; 1. Because they understood and were a really good friend,

2. They were scared of me and what I was capable of if they challenged me, or 3. One and Two combined.

Relationships: Sink or Swim

I bet you thought this last one would be about sex, right? Nah, sex during pregnancy and whether it is off the charts HOT, average as can be or less than mediocre, it's specific to your body and your circumstance, but relationships, now THAT is something to talk about!

I always heard that having a baby is similar to planning a wedding in terms of whether relationships in your life will survive or not, and I have to say, YES THAT IS SO TRUE OH MY GOD!

In less dramatic terms, planning for a baby challenges most if not all relationships in your life. Your emotional state goes through transition and adjustment. Your ability to do things you used to do is compromised temporarily, and sometimes permanently. It's a time where you need the support of your family and friends, and as a result, sometimes they show up, and sometimes they don't.

It's quite an eye-opening experience to go through an entire pregnancy and then be a new mother and STILL maintain the same relationships. If you can do that without loss, then you're probably one of the lucky few. But I wouldn't quite say that it's unlucky to lose people you thought were your friends during this process. Like planning a wedding, preparing for a baby is just another life event that weeds out the superficial relationships from the ones that will always be there, and to me, that's an absolute bonus of pregnancy.

Sure, pregnancy has its cons, its downfalls and its (FUCK THIS SHIT I'M NEVER DOING THIS AGAIN) moments, but it can be amazing, and enjoyable and pleasantly surprising. With both pregnancies I was pleasantly blown away by not only how much I loved being pregnant, but how well I did it and how much I'll always want to do it again. But Fuck No!

PREGNANCY SYMPTOMS THAT YOU WILL HATE!

RACHEL SOBEL

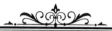

> *"Pregnancy is a simultaneously beautiful, disgusting,*
> *mind-blowing, exhausting, terrifying, miraculous,*
> *and surreal journey. Pause every so often to remember*
> *the moments along the way."*
> *- Whine and Cheez-its*

"Having my wisdom teeth out was far more painful than childbirth."

That's the first lie someone told me when I was pregnant with my first child. The person was my mother.

Women (at least my tribe) typically overshare many details of their lives. We cover everything from diet to bra size to sex and everything in between. However, all bets are off when it comes to pregnancy. Sure, veteran preggos shared some highs and lows with me, but NOTHING prepared me for the reality of what pregnancy does to your mind, body, and soul. While nobody flat out lied (well, except my mother), there were MANY lies by omission.

A LOT.

With my first, I was blissfully ignorant going in. Like a blank, knocked-up canvas. I peed on the stick, got a little plus sign, ordered a famous pregnancy book and subscribed to the app that equates your baby's size to that of some obscure produce like an English hothouse cucumber or a kumquat. My overall pregnancy knowledge was intricately linked to those two sources. Each week I would read about what was happening to my body, in very clinical (read conservative) terms, and simultaneously learn about my baby's development.

That's where it ended, so that's what I knew.

Well, let me tell you something…. the stuff that is NOT in the books and apps is what blew my mind and endured with no warning whatsoever. So, I made it my mission among my sisterhood to spread the good word. The truth. When asked the question, "So what is Pregnancy like," I would reply with, "Do you want the REAL truth, or do you want me to regurgitate the stuff you read in books?"

If they opt for the former, I dig in and give them a dose of what to really expect, in the way I wish someone would have for me. It's like a crash course in the parts of pregnancy nobody wants to talk about, but I'm not scared.

I think the best place to start is at the top, literally.

What's That Smell?!?

You now have a superpower you never wanted – the ability to smell everything before anyone else around you notice it, if at all. You smell your husband's used coffee cup in the sink, your other kid's fart in the next room and the fish your neighbor is cooking three doors down. It comes out of nowhere, and once you smell it, there's no un-smelling it. You will also get immediately nauseated by seemingly innocent and mild smells that never bothered you before, like cucumbers and taco shells, for absolutely no reason. And if you are one of the lucky ones who experience morning (or all day) sickness, you'll have intermittent dry-heaving and possible puking throughout the day. I actually kept a puke bag in my purse and car just in case heaving turned to hurling.

The Gag Reflex is Strong with This One.

The mundane task of brushing your teeth now comes with a pretty significant gag reflex. You don't even have to hit the back of your throat with your toothbrush. Just brush your back molars and surprise, you're dry heaving (that's a common theme in pregnancy). Another thing you should know about the mouth and nose area – you are one hearty sneeze or cough away from peeing your pants. Might want to stick an extra pair of undies in your purse.

Speaking of Gagging.

When you already have weird aversions to smell and taste, the last thing you want to do is to chug a bottle of sugar. Enter the glucose test. During the latter part of your pregnancy, even with all of the crazy technology we have in the field of medicine, we still have to drink an archaic, overly sweet concoction and then have blood drawn (for the seventy-fifth time) to check for gestational diabetes. Since my first pregnancy, they have thankfully decreased the amount of fluid ounces and increased the flavor options, but none of them are good. It's kind of like when you were in high school and sat in someone's driveway drinking Boone's Farm, but minus the buzz.

Just Buy All the Tums.

Heartburn is one thing. Pregnancy heartburn is a whole different beast. A beast that feels like it's eating its way out of your esophagus slowly, while it breathes scorching, relentless fire along the way. You don't even have to eat or drink anything to get it, and it comes on fast leading to you popping tums like potato chips. The gas is right behind the heartburn. Pun intended.

Those Can't Be My Nipples.

Never in my life did I know how large your nipples could get and how many shades darker they could turn. And it's not a gradual change. You catch a glimpse of yourself in the mirror one day as you waddle into the shower and audibly gasp because you can't even believe they are yours and not something you might find in an issue of National Geographic.

Why Is There Hair There?

If you are super lucky, you will be the recipient of a hard-to-miss dark line that goes from your belly button down. Like all the way down. Sometimes it also extends up in the opposite direction. As if that is not awesome enough you can even grow hair around the same area. Like out of nowhere, wiry, dark hair on your midsection.

Your Vagina Is Like a Build-a-Bear.

Vaginal birth can wreak some havoc. I mean, sure, we know that the vagina can expand to allow your child to exit freely, but sometimes it's not so simple, and you need a little help in the form of an episiotomy OR a little damage control after because of tearing. Like a piece of paper out of a notebook. That means you get stitched up, just like the teddy bear your child creates from scratch in the mall as you are dipping into your life savings to purchase it and all of the clothes for it that your kid passes on the way to the register.

TBT to Your Ankles

Since parts of your body swell with no warning, you will soon have mini tree stumps where your ankles used to be, accompanied by Flintstone feet. You know what I'm talking about, those oversized, clunky hooves that don't look like they belong on your body.

Sayonara Sleep

About a million people will tell you that the reason you have such a hard time sleeping during pregnancy is that your body is getting you ready for the tremendous sleep deficit you will experience as a new parent. If you ask me, it's because you feel like a beached whale with nowhere to go. As your belly grows so does the discomfort. You can't sleep on your back. Stomach sleepers are screwed. And the safe place known as side sleeping is a fleeting comfort, as you have to keep switching sides because the leg underneath you goes numb. You end up propping yourself up with a ton of pillows, and binge-watching Vanderpump Rules at 3 am while adding clever graphic onesies to your online shopping cart for your child who isn't even here yet.

This doesn't even scratch the surface of things that can happen during pregnancy. We haven't even delved into uncomfortable internal exams, sex, and bodily fluids. Not even a little. But you have to start somewhere, and at the very least it lays a good foundation to help alleviate the shock and awe of what happens to your body when you are growing a human.

Despite everything from the lack of sleep right down to the cankles, it's worth every single hush- hush detail of pregnancy. Maybe just maybe, more women will start to share the good, bad AND ugly just as easily as your one know-it-all mom friend doles out unsolicited advice on parenting.

PREGNANCY SYMPTOMS THAT MIGHT SCARE YOU!

HOLLY LOFTIN

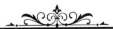

> *"Sit back, relax, and enjoy the bumpy ride. The best thing you can do is stay positive and milk every pregnancy symptom for all it's worth. Just remember, after this baby is born, it will never be about YOU again."*
> *-From the Bottom of My Purse*

Some women absolutely love pregnancy. They feel amazing, only gain fifteen pounds, and have soft, glowing skin, like a newborn's bottom. Then there's me; who had any, and all pregnancy ailments that an expectant mother can have, and then some. I'm not even talking about simple, ordinary things, like morning sickness, relentless back pain, and looking like a beached-whale from all angles. I mean, I had all those symptoms too, but what I'm talking about is the uncommon crap they fail to warn a girlfriend about in those buttoned-up pregnancy books. The rare things, that if they happen with your first pregnancy, you most likely will not procreate again. Lucky for me, all this happened with my second, and final, pregnancy.

God sure does have an odd sense of humor.

These horrendous pregnancy symptoms have remained hush-hush for long enough. Many women are going into pregnancy blindly, expecting ten months (I don't ever say nine, because let's be honest, that's a bunch of BS) of pure bliss, where they roll around in Cheetos and get waited on hand and foot. I'm here to save you a lot of pain, suffering, and incessant calls to the OBGYN. Ok, that's a lie, you will still need your OBGYN on speed dial, but at least you won't be calling your husband frantically telling him that you think you are "dying."

I'm not trying to scare you or say any of this will happen to you, because, chances are, none of this will happen to you. I'm pretty sure that most women have the "perfect, uneventful pregnancy" that you see portrayed all over social media, but on the off-chance, you are dealt a shit sandwich like I was, and experience some of these phenomena, at least you will know that you're not alone and that you will survive. I got your back.

So listen up, ladies.....

Bleeding doesn't always mean something is wrong with the baby.

When you see blood during pregnancy, your mind immediately goes dark, but sometimes women bleed during pregnancy for no known reason. And they can bleed a lot. I had something called a Subchorionic Hemorrhage, which sounds scary AF, but after a lot of late night Google searches I found it isn't that uncommon. It happens when a blood clot forms between the uterus and the placenta and causes bleeding.

This happened to me when I was nine weeks pregnant, and naturally, I was in a tailspin. I had never heard of such a thing, but when I started telling people about it, I got a lot of "Oh yeah, I had a friend of a friend that had that too, and everything turned out just fine." Why the heck are people not talking about this? It's like some secret pregnancy society where women are bleeding and never speaking a word about it. It scared the crap out of me, and a head's up would've been nice. So try to remain calm if you see blood. Blood doesn't always mean miscarriage. In fact, more than 50% of the time, bleeding doesn't mean miscarriage. The odds are in your favor. You should always still consult with your doctor, on the off chance it is something more serious.

You may leak fluid.

When you see your underwear soaked at twenty weeks, you immediately think something is very wrong. This happened to me, and I was rushed to Labor and Delivery to get examined and test the fluid because they suspected it was amniotic fluid. I remember the doctor came in to talk to me about how if it was amniotic fluid, there was "nothing they could do," and I would most likely lose the baby. It was gut-wrenching and beyond terrifying. Waiting in that sterile room for the test results was the longest hour of my life. I wouldn't wish that upon my worst enemy.

After the results came back, they determined that it was "just urine," not amniotic fluid. So basically, I was peeing on myself in large quantities. I was so elated that everything was OK; I didn't even care that the entire Labor and Delivery Unit knew I needed to wear Depends. I continued to piss myself the remainder of my pregnancy because my beautiful bundle decided to camp out on my bladder and do summersaults twenty-four seven, but it was all good; I survived. Pregnancy is very humbling at times.

Your hormones may go crazy.

I knew that I would be an emotional basket case and do outlandish things, like burst into tears during a Hallmark commercial or go postal on the barista at Starbucks because she put "whip" instead of "no-whip" (hypothetically speaking, of course). But what I didn't know is that I could get issues like an overactive thyroid and anemia. I remember feeling so worn down that I had to force myself to get out of bed and care for my five-year-old. Just slathering peanut butter and jelly on his crustless bread took all the energy I had. I chalked it up to pregnancy and just pressed on, but I wish I had listened to my body sooner.

If you feel like complete and utter crap and can barely function, have your doctor check your hormone levels. You should be exhausted during pregnancy, but not being able to get out of the bed or take a shower usually means there is something bigger going on. It's such an easy fix once you get diagnosed. The thyroid medicine started to reduce symptoms almost immediately, and iron levels usually increase within a month. Don't suffer in silence.

You may have low blood pressure.

Every pregnant woman is warned about the dangers of high blood pressure and risks of preeclampsia, but what if you have low blood pressure? I know that low blood pressure is ideal in theory, but when you are carrying a life inside of you and have a blood pressure of 88/50, you feel like complete and utter poop. I remember pleading with my doctor to do something, because "I could not go on like this," and he kept advising me to load up on salt and drink plenty of water. I don't know if you've experienced constant morning sickness, the kind where you are praying to the porcelain throne twenty-four seven, but the last thing you want to do is load up on salt and water. Eventually, they agreed to give me regular IV fluids, and the difference was night and day.

Sometimes, you have to throw your weight (you're larger than life preggo weight) around at the OBGYN's office. Don't worry; they are used to outlandish requests and hostile women. They chose this profession. If your blood pressure is low, and you feel like you're going to pass out every time you stand, and your doctor is dismissing you—demand treatment. I felt like I could run a marathon the days I got fluids.

Please don't think that any of this stuff is the norm. Pregnancy is a blissful experience for many women. I have friends who loved being pregnant and didn't experience one single symptom. Damn them! At the end of the day, after all the pain and suffering, I would do it all over again, one million times. The day I held my beautiful daughter in my arms, I forgot every wretched thing from the past ten months. Pregnancy amnesia is a thing. I think a horrible pregnancy mentally prepares us to embrace the fact that our life is "no longer ours any more" and that we will be bitching and moaning for the next eighteen years anyway. Lean in, ladies. Motherhood is painful AF.

Pregnancy Story Time

DURING PREGNANCY, PUKE HAPPENS. TAKE ADVICE WITH A GRAIN OF SALTINE.

KAREN LESH

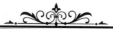

"Eat what you want, but definitely try crackers."
- MOB Truths

We all have those friends who were "so nauseous" in their first trimester, but who never threw up, and who simply felt better after "a glass of water and some fruit." You know . . . THOSE friends.

I am not that friend. If I've done the math right, I threw up close to 2,000 times over the course of my three pregnancies. Yes, really. TWO. THOUSAND.

How is that even possible? Well, name a place – any place. I puked there. Kitchen sink? Yes. Home Depot parking lot? You bet. Side yard of my house? Yes. Restaurant bathroom, office trash can (not the bathroom, but the trash can at my actual desk), shower, plastic bag in a car, hotel bathroom in the US, Argentina, and Germany, airport bathroom, bathroom at home, Target parking lot, doctor's office . . . You get the idea.

Yes, spontaneous upchucking became so routine for me that I remember asking my husband during my first pregnancy, "Was there ever a time when I didn't throw up first thing in the morning? I honestly don't remember what those days were like."

Pregnancy is an amazing, beautiful state of being, or at least that's how I viewed it and how I felt, despite the fact that I always had to stash plastic bags in my glove compartment or laptop bag or coat pocket just in case. I reasoned that all this puking was a sign of dramatic hormonal stuff going on in my body as it crafted an entire human being in there. Pretty wondrous stuff.

For me, each of the three pregnancies differed . . . Except for the one striking similarity of seemingly constant vomiting. Amidst all the uncertainty and questioning that goes on during pregnancy, one thing is certain: I did everything I could think of to feel better. Wouldn't you if you were throwing up randomly, multiple times a day, for almost 9 months at a time?

Did anything help me? Sure, I found lots of remedies, but each one seemed to work for only a few weeks and then wear off. Popsicles, even in the middle of the night. Water with a splash of lemonade mix. Pizza – yes, pizza! Pancakes (until I once puked them up in the kitchen sink because I couldn't get to the bathroom fast enough). Lollipops. Pretzels. French fries. Oranges. I had a long list of remedies that would work for a few weeks at a time and then – boom – one day they'd stop working, and I'd have to find something else.

Countless articles and social media posts have been written about the hilarious, though often frustrating, unwelcome advice pregnant women receive about just about everything. "Don't wear high heels," a colleague in my office used to tell me. "Don't paint your nails – the chemicals can harm the baby." "Eat this not that, and never those . . ." You know what I'm talking about. And all the judgy questions! "You're pregnant already? Didn't you just get married?" Or "You're pregnant again? Didn't you just have a baby?" or "What if it's another boy?" (It was!).

And if you're "lucky" like I was and felt noticeably sick or frequently engaged in sudden public vomiting (I swear I tried to be discreet, but it didn't always work!), the advice came flowing in. Ginger, ginger tea, real ginger tea ... the fancy lollipops that are intended to help nausea ... more water . . . Exercise. . . Less exercise . . . You must not be eating enough. .you have to keep eating even if you're sick because the baby needs the nutrients...

Luckily my doctors were savvy and knowledgeable and most of all, human. They reassured me that the baby takes the nutrients he needs from me, and as long as he was growing fine and I was keeping weight on, the vomiting was more of an inconvenience than a real issue.

"How far along are you? I'm sure you'll feel better once you're done with the first trimester."

I didn't.

Of all the unsolicited advice I received about how to manage my pregnancy nausea and vomiting, my favorite by far, was this simple, well-intentioned statement: "Have you tried eating some crackers before getting out of bed in the morning?"

"OH, CRACKERS?" I had been throwing up for 19 weeks, and these people didn't think I'd thought of CRACKERS yet? Like almost 5 months had gone by with me forcefully spewing contents out of my gut, up to and including bile, and I hadn't tried a delicious yet superbly bland and comforting SALTINE yet? Seriously, people? Crackers? Of course, I've tried *@$^##%*crackers!

What's the point of all this? To warn you, to reassure you, and hopefully to make you smile. Pregnancy is an amazing but wacky journey, full of unimaginable physical and emotional changes, and a LOT of unsolicited advice. I'd like to think that handling most of it with grace was imprinted on my three baby boys when each was born . . . But that remains to be seen. Yeah, my crackers reaction was snarky any time someone approached me with that suggestion, but I was entitled, I think. And if you know me, you know that my "snarky" still often sounds like other people's Mickey Mouse/sweetheart tones. But in case it was taken the wrong way, I hereby apologize for snapping at anyone who mentioned Saltines, and I challenge you to find a new, creative remedy for puking while pregnant.

In the meantime, I have three healthy, happy, utterly silly rascal boys who brighten my day every day. And when they misbehave, I merely remind them I puked my brains out for 9 months for each of them while growing them in my belly. Respect. I deserve it.

DURING PREGNANCY, CRAP HAPPENS. IT HELPS TO HAVE A SENSE OF HUMOR.

BRITT LEBOEUF

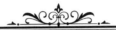

> *"From the moment that double line appears you are a Mama. Whether you carry your baby for one day or go full term, a part of your soul has been awakened that can never be dormant again."*
> *–These Boys of Mine*

Pregnancy is a beautiful thing. The idea that we get to carry the loves of our lives in our bodies still amazes me! Although it's beautiful, thrilling and exciting, it can also be gross, painful, and embarrassing.

I had a textbook pregnancy with my first son. However, my pregnancy with my second son was awful! I had nausea in the first trimester, my weight gain was more so than it was in my other pregnancy, and the heartburn I suffered from was almost unbearable! It was not fun! I was always complaining to my husband. Let's say neither of us could wait for the pregnancy to be over with!

The icing on the cake was one day when we traveled a couple of towns over to get groceries at a store that was quieter than our usual grocery store. We enjoyed the ride across the county; it was filled with farms, pine forests and stretches of land with nobody around for miles. It was the end of the summer, so I was about six months along at that point. After we got our groceries, we decided to get some lunch at the local Chinese buffet. I had eaten at this restaurant dozens of times in the past; it is home to the best Chinese food in our area. What pregnant lady doesn't love a buffet? I ate for two that day! We paid our bill, made one last stop at another store and then started on the forty-five minute ride home through the mostly unpopulated part of our county.

As I drove us home, my husband was sitting next to me in the passenger seat, and we were discussing the latest episode of "The Walking Dead." That's when it hit me. A wave of heat came over me as if someone had suddenly cranked the heat of my tiny car. It was almost like how our moms describe their hot flashes. Although it was a warm summer day, we had the air conditioning on, and I hadn't been sweating just two minutes prior. Next, came the gurgling. I could hear and feel my stomach working on some kind of voodoo deep inside the confines of my abdomen.

My husband seemed oblivious as he continued to talk about Rick Grimes and company. I started to panic as I felt the first twinge of pressure down there. I had to poop! And I had to poop now!

"I think I have to go to the bathroom," I said as I interrupted my husband's chatter. He just looked at me with a surprised look on his face and said, "Like you have to pee?"

I shook my head no. He now knew the severity of the situation. "Can you hold it for a little while?" He asked. I started to squirm. I knew that it wasn't going to wait for very long. The need to find a toilet was imminent and immediately necessary.

"We are in the middle of nowhere," he said, only adding to my list of problems. Then an idea came over his face. "My uncle's land is up the road a little ways here. They have the camp at the end of the dirt road with an outhouse. Can you make it that far?" he asked.

I hadn't thought of the camp. I had been there a few times in the past but never in this dire of a situation. It would have to do. I didn't respond to him I just stepped on the gas, praying I'd make it to the camp in time. With each new stretch of road that appeared before us, I could feel myself fighting off the urge to go to the bathroom.

"I can't crap my pants," I shouted out loud finally to break the silence and distract myself from what was happening. My husband, always the calm and collected one just held my hand and said, "We're close." A couple of turns down the desolate road later and we squealed into the gravel parking lot that leads to the dirt road to the camp. As I climbed out of the car, I remembered we had just bought toilet paper on our grocery run. I reached into the back seat and grabbed a roll and then started hightailing it towards the camp.

As I was trying to hold everything in, I was also in an extreme start of anxiety as the grass on the side of the road was long, and my husband had seen several snakes on it in the past. I am terrified of snakes! So here I was, six months pregnant, trying to keep myself from pooping my pants in the middle of nowhere, and on the lookout for snakes on the road. Thankfully my husband took the lead and was looking down at the ground as we walked.

The walk to the camp felt like it took one hundred years. I was in a battle with my body that I knew I was not going to win for much longer. Finally, as we rounded the corner of the dirt road, I could see the outhouse in the distance. It was located in the woods next to the camp.

When we were within six feet of the outhouse door, my body betrayed me. As hard as I tried, I couldn't hold it in any longer. Just as my husband reached for the door and opened it for me, I started to crap my pants. I could feel it hit the back of my pants and get warm down the back of my legs. As I entered the outhouse, I pulled my pants down and finished what I had already started on the toilet.

It was too late. There was no going back now. For the first time since I was a child, I crapped my pants.

The small outhouse stunk to the high heavens, and I just sat there for a few minutes in complete shock and horror. My sweet husband came and knocked on the door a few minutes later. "Are you okay in there?" he asked.

"I didn't make it in time," I stated matter-of-factly.

He knew better than to respond. I asked him to get my purse from the car as well as my jacket out of the back. While I waited for him to returns with my things, I cleaned myself up the best I could. Thank God I had grabbed the toilet paper because there was none in the outhouse!

I stripped myself from the waist down. When my husband came back, he handed me my things through the semi-open door. I chucked my underwear in the outhouse toilet, they were a lost cause, through my capris in the grocery bag my husband had thought to bring me, and tied my jacket around my waist.

I walked back to my car like this. Thankfully the road was mostly deserted, and the way I had parked didn't allow for any passing vehicles to see anything anyways. I was covered in all the right places though. My husband got into the driver's seat because I was too mortified to drive. He didn't say anything about it the entire ride home. He knew I didn't want to talk about it.

When we got back home, I immediately ran upstairs and jumped into the shower. When I came back downstairs, my husband had put the groceries away and was sitting at the kitchen table. That's when we started to laugh. He was sworn to secrecy and told me it had even happened to him a couple of times as an adult after he had eaten something that didn't agree with him.

We both agreed it must have been something I had eaten at the restaurant that either the baby or my body didn't like. Although I didn't quite make it to the toilet that day, I'll never forget how gracious and kind my husband was in that situation. I'll always be grateful that I had toilet paper in my car and my jacket stashed in my trunk.

For you, momma-to-be, I recommend you always bring an extra set of pants! You may not think this could happen to you, but it can. Trust me, I never thought I'd crap my pants as an adult, but hey, it happened.

THE ITCHY PREGNANCY

MEAGAN HALTIWANGER

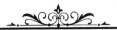

> *"Trust your body, even when it's terrifying and painful.*
> *And trust the love that's coming. It's a love so pure and true,*
> *you won't understand how you lived without it before."*
> *- Life of Owen*

Sometimes we want to know others stories, so we know that we are not alone. Often our google search results tend to bring more fear than comfort. In my journey of pregnancy and motherhood, I have found that knowing a personal connection can help transform my often irrational fears to comfort. Knowing someone on the other side of an experience gives us the courage, strength and hope to believe that we might make it to the other side too. Looking back, I wish I had known someone else who had experienced a bizarre pregnancy story like mine.

I met many women along those long, drawn out, never-ending nine months who were nauseated, puking, insomniacs, cranky, fill-in-the-blank with another symptom. And believe me, I don't discount those symptoms at all. I threw up every day until the day my son was born, and then while in labor I threw up seventy-two times. Yup, seventy-two puking sessions in a forty hour labor with a four-hour pushing session that ended in an emergency C-section. My doula said she had never seen anything like it. But labor was by no means the worst of my pregnancy journey.

I cried all the time while pregnant. I was anxious often. So anxious in fact that one of my fears was that I would be taken to the psychiatric ward and stuck there until he was born (I wish I were kidding). I could go on and on. Truthfully, I don't believe that one symptom is any easier than others. If you are hurting or scared or sick, it doesn't matter the cause. Every symptom and fear and pain is miserable. It's just that the symptom

I had the last trimester was so unusual I felt like a complete pariah. And I was terrified. Because I had never met anyone who itched like I did during their pregnancy.

The itching started at Owen's baby shower in Alabama. I had been looking forward to the day for months. My mom was in town from Hawaii, and I just wanted to feel happy about a pregnancy that had been challenging. The pregnancy had drained me thus far, and it felt more like an awful nightmare than the blissful, joyful experience I had originally dreamed it to be. As the baby shower began, I was able to relax and stay in the moment. I was huge (my son ended up being nine lbs. nine oz.) and could barely move at that point, but I was so grateful to be surrounded by so much love.

As the shower was winding down, I started to notice my arm felt extra itchy. I sweat a lot anyway, and at one thousand pounds pregnant, I was a sweaty, broken faucet that wouldn't stop leaking. I initially blamed it on the heat. Owen's baby shower was in May in Alabama. Surely the rash on my arms had to be from the heat and nerves from the shower, right?

We left the shower and headed home. Somehow the rash had crawled its way through my skin to my other arm. But I was focused on the adorable baby clothes and gifts we had received. I didn't even think to be worried about this weird, sudden rash. For the remainder of the weekend, I focused on enjoying time with my mom and setting up the nursery. By the time she left on Sunday, things had taken a sudden turn for the worse.

The rash was spreading and growing in size. My legs started swelling with welts, and my body felt as if I had rolled around in poison ivy. It looked like it too. I called the on-call doctor, and they called in a steroid for me for the next day until they could see me in person. They told me I was safe to take Benadryl that evening, so I went to bed hoping for some Benadryl-induced sleep.

It was a Monday morning when I went to go pick up the medication from the pharmacy. I took off from school (I was an elementary gifted teacher at the time) and drove myself to the pharmacy. By this point, the rash had spread to my stomach as well. The doctor was going to see me later in the day, but until then thought the medicine would ease the symptoms. I was miserable and so confused on what was happening to my body. I quickly grabbed the medication from the local CVS and headed home. But I didn't quite make it home.

The CVS was less than two miles from my house in Homewood, Alabama. But I had to cross a busier intersection to get back into my neighborhood. And with lack of sleep and major discomfort from all the itching, I wasn't in the most alert state to be driving. I pulled out to cross and was immediately hit on the driver's side by a car coming much faster than I had anticipated. He missed my door by mere inches. I was thirty-two weeks pregnant, and my large belly slammed into the steering wheel with an immense amount of force.

I panicked. What if Owen was hurt? I couldn't feel him moving and was terrified that something was wrong. The man immediately jumped out of his car to talk to me. I didn't move. He began chastising me for being so careless, but as soon as he saw how pregnant I was, he stopped in his tracks. He called 911, and others stopped to help. I remember a woman talking to me telling me it was all going to be okay. I was so scared. I called Owen's dad and told him what happened and which hospital to meet me at. I didn't seem to be too severely injured on the outside. But no one had any idea about Owen.

They rushed me to the hospital by ambulance. Unfortunately, they did not have any fetal monitors within the ambulance. That ride was agonizing, not knowing whether my baby was okay or not. My blood pressure was majorly elevated, and they kept telling me to try and stay calm to not induce labor. Once we arrived at the hospital, they immediately hooked me up to a monitor to hear his heartbeat. We heard the thump, thump sound of his sweet little heart. And with the biggest sigh of relief, we knew he was fine.

There are certain moments of life that I feel like are part of our stories that we forever remember, moments that become so deeply embedded within us it's hard to remember a time before those moments. My accident with Owen is one of my moments.

But even more so was what happened after. My rash progressed. The word PUPPS was mentioned, a word I had never heard before. When the doctor finally saw me, she told me she had never seen a case quite like mine. PUPPS stands for a fancy, long-winded name that means you develop a hive-like rash that lasts until the birth of your baby, if not longer. The good news is that it does not harm the baby. The bad news is that it is the most uncomfortable, frustrating health issue because there is nothing to be done about it but stay uncomfortable and wait.

I thought I would feel so much relief and joy that Owen was fine after the accident. And believe me, I did. But I also felt insane, because I itched all the time. I scratched so often that I would bleed. Years later, I still have scars. I took oatmeal baths. I use Grandpa's Old Pine Tar Soap three times a day. I ate dandelion capsules. I took steroids. I used every cream and lotion available. My mom even ordered me a special kind of oil from Australia that claimed to help specifically with PUPPS. I would find relief for a few minutes at most and then the itching would resume.

I lived the last two months of my pregnancy alternating between scratching and crying. I read horror stories of moms who continued to have symptoms for months, if not years after their baby was born. I was terrified I would never feel like myself again. PUPPS took a major toll on me not only physically, but also mentally. But finally, five days after his due date, Owen arrived. And with his arrival, my PUPPS disappeared. It took some time, but my body slowly began to heal. To say I was grateful and relieved was an understatement. Through Owen's pregnancy and other major life events, I have learned that much of what happens in life is entirely out of our control. Sometimes all we can do is take some Benadryl and hope for the best.

PREGNANCY IS ALL THE RAGE

BIANCA JAMOTTE LEROUX

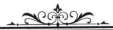

> *"Write down your very detailed birth plan and then burn it, nothing will go according to plan EVER again, and that's ok."*
> *- Real Mommy Confessions*
>
> **"I know this isn't you talking, it's your hormones, but I would just like to say fuck you, hormones. You are a crazy bitch, hormones. Hormones, fuck 'em!"**
> **~ Seth Rogan as Ben Stone, Knocked Up**

I was surprised by how steady my mood had been throughout my pregnancy. I think this was due, in part, to how excited I was to be pregnant. I was having my long-awaited daughter and entered my second trimester feeling fantastic. My belly was swollen, but I felt strong and sexy. My skin was clear (we'll say I was glowing, but as it was New York in the middle of summer, it was probably just sweat). I was cute and pregnant and loving every second of it.

We lived in Brooklyn at the time, just down the street from the coffee shop my husband and I own which I had worked in every morning until I was too big to stand comfortably behind the small counter.

I spent most of my summer days walking around our neighborhood, hanging out at the coffee shop with our regulars, and enjoy my changing body and life. I may be the only woman on the planet who enjoyed strangers touching my baby bump; I loved attention from the old Polish women in our neighborhood. We didn't speak the same language, but we pieced together a universal language of motherhood.

The florist around the corner would give me fresh cut flowers as I passed his shop, and the young women dressed in 1950s-style mint green uniforms behind the counter at the donut shop snuck extra donuts into my bag. I felt cared for by everyone I met. And then I entered my third trimester. I expected there would be significant changes in my hormone levels, but nothing prepared me (or Brooklyn) for the mood swings I experienced as my body prepared for birth.

I missed my family in California, my baby shower was being held on my 30th birthday and somehow became something I had to plan for myself, and I was feeling alone and scared. The slightest thing would make me cry. I figured I would spend my final month sobbing while cleaning the pantry for the sixth time.

I was getting bigger by the minute and had started waddling more than walking. As my stomach continued to grow, so did my false sense of invincibility. There was the time a woman insulted my dog, and I lost my shit. My landlord grabbed my arm as I stepped off the curb to confront her and defend my dog's honor. Did I care that I was thirty-two weeks pregnant? Nope; I knew I could take her. That woman was lucky she was on the other side of the street.

By September I had given in and started driving everywhere I needed to go. New York drivers were not kind to me. I took personally every glare and honk each time I tried driving into the city and ended up calling my husband crying while crossing one of the bridges to get home.

Once, while I was stuck behind a truck, a man in Brooklyn kept honking at me, even though I couldn't move my car. We got out of our vehicles—he, a fat, middle-aged man, and me, the obviously pregnant thirty-year-old woman—and I challenged him to "Come at me!" I hadn't thought through what he would do, but my pregnancy hormones told me I could handle just about anything.

I wish I could say this was the only time road rage got the best of me.

One day, as I was driving home down one of the main avenues in a trendy neighborhood in Brooklyn, I was cut off by a driver in a fancy white car with crazy rims that looked like there was spinning in three different directions at the same time. Uncharacteristically for my third trimester, I took a deep breath and kept driving steadily forward. But then the driver stuck his arm out of the window flipped me off and honked at me. He cut me off, and he was rude to me?!

"OH FUCK, NO!"

I yelled this to myself as I slammed my foot on the accelerator pedal and started weaving in and out of traffic chasing him down. He made a quick right, and I started laughing maniacally because this was MY 'HOOD. I knew he had just turned down a street that has a stoplight at every intersection. He was definitely going to get stuck.

I turned down a side road and sped to see if I could cut him off at the pass.

I was right; he was stopped at the red as I made the turn in front of his car, crossed over the double yellow line into oncoming traffic, and parked my big soon-to-be-mommy-mobile perpendicular to his vehicle in the intersection. I swung open my door and waddled quickly to his window, screaming at him, "How dare you treat people so badly?! You think it's okay to drive like a crazy person and then flip ME off like it was my fault?!"

He rolled down his dark window and stared at my face angrily. Then his eyes slowly made their way down to my swollen belly, and he started laughing.

My heart began to race, and I could hear my pulse in my ears as my body flushed hot with rage. His painted and push-up bra-wearing girlfriend started laughing, he waved his big hairy arm at me and finally said, "Get back in your car, crazy pregnant lady." He attempted to roll up his black window, but I wasn't finished.

I put my hand on his window and leaned in closer. But instead of looking at him, I spoke to his girlfriend.

"You. You should pick better men. You're very pretty and could do way better than this asshole."

I turned quickly and waddled back to my car, slammed my door, and sped off. By the time I drove past the end of the block, my adrenaline had started crashing, and reality set it. Humiliation from the scene I had just caused made me feel hot and numb like all the blood was draining from my body. I called my husband (who was furious with me for putting myself in danger), and carefully drove home as he talked me down.

Thankfully, I went into labor three weeks early.

Once I held my beautiful baby girl, I was instantly changed, I was a mother, her mother. I had never loved the smell, the feel, the weight of anything as much as I adored my daughter. The next few days were a blur of bonding and settling into my new role. My hormones returned to normal; or, at least, as normal as I could have hoped.

And then…

My Momma Bear instincts kicked in. I shouted at a complete stranger as my husband dragged me out of the bagel shop. "Who the hell thinks it's a good idea to ask a mother if her infant has a fucking overbite?"

I THOUGHT I KNEW

STACEY WALTZER

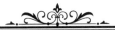

> *"Go ahead and register for a powerful Dust buster.*
> *Trust me…One day you will understand."*
> *~ 40 Wishes and Counting*

Everything about babies fascinated me when I was a kid. I had many dolls in my bedroom that I pretended were real. Dressing them up, rocking them to sleep, and even taking one out for a walk in my cabbage patch stroller convinced me that being a mommy was my calling. One day, I announced to my mom that I was going to have nineteen babies.

To her credit, she didn't laugh right into my face. She tried to walk away as her laughter trailed behind her. I had no clue what was so funny. Of course at that age, I had no concept of mom life or even how to make a baby.

When I was old enough to figure things out, I still thought I would become a mom, but there was no way I was having that many kids! Who could afford them? Where would all of us live? This was still long before you could make a fortune off being a hit show about life with so many babies.

Years later, all of my dreams changed.

It was while I was at a very good friend's house babysitting for their two little ones. The kids had gone to bed, and I saw a copy of a very famous pregnancy book. Thinking it would be interesting to flip through, I started to read.

Hours later, I wished I never picked it up. By the time my friends got home, I was traumatized. They found me on a chair in a state of disbelief with lots of questions.

Vaginal discharge?

Nosebleeds?

THE BELLY BUTTON POPS OUT??? How does that even work? Do you feel something like that?

What are hemorrhoids?

Varicose veins, breasts swelling and spotting. This is pregnancy? The shock was building.

Then it got to the actual birth. After figuring out how the exact size of ten centimeters, I was done.

I declared I would not be having babies after all.

But something inside me felt different some more years later after getting married and seeing other friends have babies. I wanted one so much that the book became a faraway memory.

My focus turned to all things Pinterest. In other words, only perfection. It would be about the cute clothes, decorating the nursery, and wearing all the amazing maternity clothes. I would register for all things awesome and carry the most stylish diaper bag. Pregnancy and being a mom would be an incredible experience.

The time came when I got pregnant and made my announcement at work where I was a teacher.

It was the year that people were warned not to drink the water in our school. It seemed everywhere you turned, there was a pregnant teacher walking by. Seven of us were expecting babies. Some were already out with their newborns.

The principal had charts up in the office with due dates and plans for maternity leaves. It was almost like an epidemic of sorts.

The expecting moms would show off sonogram pictures. Each week someone would be talking about a different fruit or vegetable that the baby was the size of. Notes would be compared on what we could have and couldn't have. I declared my doctor was the best as I walked around with the one cup of coffee I was allowed to have.

Things became more real as my stomach got bigger. I learned how to make my pants last longer with a hair tie. Who knew maternity underwear existed? Not me and when I did figure out postpartum that all mine had stretched, I wished I did! The one bathroom in the hallway wasn't enough anymore as all the babies seemed to sit on our bladders at the same time.

Yet we glowed and were still caught up in the excitement. That's when things started to happen that brought the book all back to me.

I had not bought or borrowed a pregnancy book. I preferred my weekly happy emails from some random website that didn't make everything seem so terrifying.

Yes, I did spot. At what point does one worry? Me from the moment I saw it which happened to be late at night when there is no nurse line to call and get feedback. I did what any person would do. I texted 100 of my closest friends who had been through this before. Learning that a drop is nothing, I took it upon myself to share this with everyone the next day ignoring the strange stares I got in return.

While I was sitting around waiting for my belly button to pop out, us pregnant teachers would compare ankle sizes. No one told us that they would swell to the point that they could combust at any minute.

Now that we were much further along, it was time for tests. During pregnancy, you are given a timeline of a variety of screenings for you and the baby to determine how you are both doing.

The baby's measurements will be updated. You will wonder how something so big is fitting inside you. Then while looking in the mirror realize exactly how when you see the size you have become. And seriously, are those breasts now going to feed an army of babies?

The glucose test was another big one. If you failed this, your entire pregnancy diet had to change. No more fun stuff for you and really when you think about it, what fun would being pregnant be? After seeing my friend not pass and what she had to cut out of her diet, led me to binge eat Girl Scout cookies the week before my test. This was just in case I had the same results and couldn't eat them for the remainder of my pregnancy. At that point, it sounded like a life sentence.

You also got to find out the position of where your baby's head was just by a doctor poking around. Who knew? My husband practically passed out at that and is still recovering on some level.

The pregnant teachers carried on. And by carried on, we were hitting the final trimesters. Baby showers were being thrown, car seats set up, names chosen and kept secret.

All we had to do at that point was wait.

When you are pregnant, one quickly learns it will never go according to "plan." The chart that hung on our principal's wall had a lot of cross-outs and rewriting. Due dates are not set in stone. People started to have their babies out of order leaving the rest of us to wonder when it would be our turn.

Then one day, I thought I knew.

It was teacher appreciation week. My desk was filled with all things chocolate and sweet. Thanks to my passing glucose test, I was happily eating all of it. The flowers of the most beautiful kind were given in a vase handed to me by a student.

Teachers these days never sit at a desk anymore but there I was because nowhere in any of my weekly emails did it say you may feel like there is a knife in your vagina as you walk so I would sit and teach. Slowly, I got up to get something, and that's when I felt the water going down the side of my leg.

Do not panic. Do NOT panic. DO NOT PANIC.

And then I panicked.

I lined up the class as we made our way down the hallway where I popped my head into every room that had a teacher mom or a pregnant teacher asking them to look and determine what I needed to do. Someone took my class, and another told me to call my doctor. I hightailed waddled it back down to my room where I went to reach for my phone. That's when what happened became clear. The vase had tipped over onto the side and water was coming off my desk and onto my chair...where I had just been sitting.

Pregnancy brain. If it was mentioned in the book, I should have been worried about that too.

Eventually, I had my baby, and everything was going well for a couple of years. That's when I made the announcement about number two which would be my next perfect pregnancy.

One would think I knew better.

IT'S OK TO DISLIKE BEING PREGNANT

HOLLY RUST

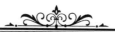

"Some of us don't GLOW during pregnancy...
instead, we look more like we won multiple pie eating
contests and pee ourselves when we sneeze."
- A Mother's Guide to Sanity

When your expectations don't meet your reality that can be a hard pill to swallow. Before having my first son, I dreamed of being pregnant. I couldn't wait to feel my baby growing inside of me. I wanted a cute baby bump. I wanted to walk through the streets rubbing my belly proudly displaying what my body could do. I wanted to love pregnancy. I tried. I really tried, but being pregnant was anything but beautiful for me.

"You're glowing. You must be so excited." People would say. No, I wasn't. I was anything but. I was excited to be a mom. I wasn't excited to continue the nine month journey of getting him here. I wanted to hold my baby in my arms. I didn't want him growing inside of me of anymore. These feelings originally came with a lot of guilt as my husband and I struggled to have our kids. We had a lot of issues and emotional ups and downs, so when it finally happened––why wasn't I happy about it? Why didn't I get all the feels that were described to me by other moms or in books I've read. I felt robbed.

About six weeks into my pregnancy, I started getting horrible vertigo. Soon after, nausea set in which hit me every night at precisely nine pm. Over the next several months, I was extremely lethargic. Every day I struggled to be grateful and tell myself it would all be worth it – but my body never came around to match those thoughts.

Of course, I had the normal complaints like peeing when I sneezed. If you're pregnant, buy yourself pads to wear now! You're welcome.

I also had insane round ligament pain that felt like rubber bands popping with each turn in bed. I had horrible congestion and bloody noses. I couldn't poop to save my life. My muscle separated from my rib, and I had sciatica. I developed hypothyroidism, which has been an ongoing battle ever since. My feet morphed into something that closely resembled bread baking in a pan that's too small for the dough. My boobs were porn star worthy but would throb with even the slightest wind gust. I'm pretty sure my husband wanted to divorce me every day for my consistent complaining. Not really, but he may have toyed with the idea. Nine months felt like two years. It may have been two years; I think we are all being lied to.

Sounds like a dream, right?

Before pregnancy, I was a working girl. I worked long hours and was always on the go. I was in the events industry, which required long nights and early mornings. My body was forcing me to slow down, which was a blessing and a curse all at the same time. It was time for me to slow down, which I didn't realize until after my son was born. My hips wouldn't work like they used to. I could no longer run to catch the train to work. I couldn't be intimate with my husband without feeling like he was doing it out of sympathy. I didn't feel like me. I wasn't me anymore. I was ashamed to talk about it because I knew there were millions of women out there who would have traded places with me in a heartbeat. I wanted this, so I had to make the best of it.

For the next few weeks, I tried to force myself to enjoy being pregnant by reading parenting books and watching A Baby Story on TV. I also signed up for pregnancy yoga and even though I made a complete fool out of myself trying to execute the moves—I enjoyed it. I met other soon-to-be moms who had the same complaints. We talked about concerns, we talked about labor, and we talked about all the things none of our other friends told us about. Thanks, jerks! Would have been nice to know about our nipples getting bigger and growing hair on our bellies before we noticed it on ourselves and freaked out! Anyway, it was nice to know I wasn't the only one who hated being pregnant and now I had a group to commiserate with.

In the midst of misery, there were a few moments of joy. The most memorable moment by far was feeling the baby's little kicks. The first time this happened, my heart nearly exploded. It's also kind of cool that you have special alone time with your baby that no one else will ever know. Listening to the heartbeat at all my doctor's appointments and finally seeing his beautiful little body growing inside of me on an ultrasound screen made the pregnancy somewhat bearable.

I couldn't wait to meet him, but mostly not be pregnant anymore. I was yearning to fall under the newborn spell, where you can't keep your hands or your lips off your new baby. When my son finally came, that dream came true and not even a week after bringing him home I told my spouse, "Let's have another!" Yes, those words actually came out of my mouth.

Did I change my thoughts about pregnancy the second time around? Absolutely not. The second time was much worse, too. The last two months I was on bed rest and had to sleep on the couch because I couldn't make it up the stairs. I convinced myself I was going into labor three different times and rushed to the hospital, only to find out my water didn't break – it was just pee. I was desperate to get him out of me because I knew what was coming. I wanted the instant love moment again; I wanted to forget what I had been going through and hold him until his feet started dragging on the floor. I knew he'd be my last, so the moment was going to be that much sweeter. And boy, did he deliver. Those baby blues still melt my heart today, and I barely remember being pregnant.

If you're someone who hates being pregnant, don't worry – you're not alone. Don't guilt yourself into thinking you should be laying in a bed of flowers spreading cocoa butter on your belly and singing lullabies to your unborn child. That's not reality. Pregnancy can be miserable; you don't have to like it. You don't have to glow. You can be annoyed by the open invitation pregnancy brings for random strangers to give you parenting advice. You don't have to smile and laugh when people ask you if you're sure if there's only one in there. In fact, I encourage you to roll your eyes. I encourage you to vent. Find a tribe and laugh together. Tell yourself every day it will be worth it. It will be worth it.

Through all the heartburn, bubble guts, leg spasms, hip pain, and watching your breasts blow up like large balloons – your body finally rewards you after a grueling nine months. You find yourself holding this little human who already recognizes your voice, gazes at you with admiration and steals your heart in less than a millisecond. The moment your baby arrives is indescribable. There are no words in the English language that can adequately describe the feeling. It's like all the pain vanishes and your mind immediately forgets what you just went through. Your heart fills up with love like you've never experienced before, and at that moment you tell yourself it was all worth it – and I promise you it is.

MY SO-CALLED AVERAGE PREGNANCY.

BROOK HALL

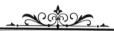

Before you have your first baby, take a moment to appreciate eating food while it is still at its desired temperature. Light candles, leave a hot cup of coffee on the table. Take a hot shower, shampoo, and condition. Shave both armpits. Go crazy. Then grab your smallest purse and spontaneously leave the house. Commit this all to memory, and you'll want to relive it in your mind in the coming months...and years.
- Stay Home Mama

My pregnancy with my first born was quite a unique experience. So many things about it were hard, scary, and unexpected, but spoiler alert: the end result was incredible. I hope my story can encourage you in some way (or at least make you watch your step more closely). If you get nothing else from this story, please know that no matter what you are going through, or have gone through, you are not alone. All our stories are different, but no "average" pregnancy is one hundred percent easy. Admitting that it is hard does not mean we aren't thankful, it does not mean we don't recognize this incredible gift we have been given, and it does not mean we don't love our babies. It simply means we are human.

I was twenty weeks pregnant, and it was the day before we were to move to a new home. My husband and I were newly married and living in an old, run-down, two-story house that had been converted into a duplex. I shudder to remember this sketchy place we lived. For example, our bathroom was in the kitchen (Super appetizing, by the way!) and only had room for one person at a time. My husband was taller than the miniature sized shower; he had to bend down to wash his hair. The stairs were narrow and short, and they were also in the kitchen. They do say the kitchen is the heart of the home, but I don't think they meant you should sit on a toilet next to the refrigerator, or run through the kitchen in a towel in order to change somewhere roomy and private. As "charming" as this place was, I was not sad to say goodbye.

On this day, I was babysitting a sweet toddler, named Kenna. She followed me around as I got ready for the day. I was dancing around the house, so thankful that it would be our last day living there. It was a chaotic mess, and there were boxes everywhere. We were upstairs looking for my hairdryer, but I couldn't find it. I picked her up and quickly hurried down the tiny stairs that led to the kitchen. As I reached the middle of the stairs, I slipped and flew down them. It happened in slow motion, and somehow, I had time to decide what to do.

Instead of trying to catch myself, I put my arms around Kenna and hugged her tight to the front of me. I fell hard onto my back, my left leg underneath me. My cell phone was upstairs, so I crawled back up the stairs while holding on to Kenna. I could feel my bones jingling, and my foot felt as though it was no longer attached to my ankle. I didn't feel any pain at first, which was a great blessing! I ended up with two broken bones in my leg and a dislocated ankle.

Eventually, I had surgery (while awake because I was pregnant) and I now have two metal plates and eight screws where my leg meets my ankle.

While recovering, unable to walk, let alone leave the house, I felt like I was missing my pregnancy. Logically, that made zero sense, it was happening inside me. I was obviously there for it, but I felt detached somehow. I wanted to be able to go out and about, showing off my baby bump, I wanted to actually wear my new maternity clothes in public, and go shopping for baby things. I couldn't use crutches because my large belly messed up my balance, so I had to use a walker or wheelchair. It's kind of a joke now, there is a walker in every picture I took of my baby bump, but I didn't find it funny at the time.

I also had kidney problems which were made much worse by my pregnancy. My left kidney was four times too big and caused an ache that wouldn't go away. If I laid flat on my back, the kidney pain was much worse, but if I tried to lay on my side, my leg would hurt worse; obviously, I couldn't lay on my stomach. The heating pad helped, but it was summer, and I was pregnant. I had to come up with creative ways to keep myself cool while also using a heating pad. I became a pro, so good in fact that I fell asleep with a heating pad on my back, it burned me and left a scar.

I remember laying on my bed watching TV and feeling so lonely. I wondered if any of the actors had ever had a broken bone. I told myself that some of them had to have suffered broken bones of some sort, and they seem perfectly fine and happy now. Even though it felt like I would be like this forever, I told myself that time WOULD go by. I would be able to get out of this bed, and this baby would come out of me and stop pressing himself into my giant kidney, everything would be okay eventually.

Friends and family helped us move the day after the incident, but my husband was working two jobs a day, which meant he was barely home, and with me practically on bed rest, we couldn't unpack. I could barely take myself to the bathroom, so going into the kitchen, making myself food, and carrying it back to my room was impossible. My husband moved the TV into our room, and I spent my days watching it on our bed alone, crying ridiculously from game shows and even commercials, laughing at myself and then crying some more.

My husband stocked my bedside table with non-perishable food and rushed home to bring me meals on his breaks from work. One day, he set the timer on the oven and forgot to turn it off before he left. I listened to the beeping for three hours before I finally got up and hopped my way through the maze of unpacked boxes to turn off the timer. I was feeling pretty good about myself, so I decided to try and make some food. I was able to pull leftover enchiladas out of the fridge and warm them up, but I spilled just outside the kitchen on the way back to my room, leaving red spots and tears on the brand-new carpet.

Another time, I wanted to do some unpacking, so I sat myself down on our computer chair and wheeled around trying to put things away. Eventually, my leg got in the way, and I ran it into a cabinet. It took me awhile, but I realized we couldn't go on this way. My husband was trying to work two jobs, care for me and take care of the household; he barely even had time to sleep. He needed some of the burdens lifted off his shoulders, and I needed company.

I finally asked for help.

My mom and her friend came over and unpacked my bedroom, which made my surroundings much less depressing. Two other friends came over and did the laundry for us, while another friend brought us food and cleaned up the kitchen. Sweet ladies from our church family brought us dinner every night for a couple of weeks. Many times, my mom brought me to their house where she could take care of me. There were also some friends who came over just to sit and hang out with me. It is amazing how knowing you're loved can make you feel miles and miles better. I realized that most people want to help, but they don't know how, and they don't want to be in the way. I have a lot of people in my life who love me and were simply waiting for me to tell them what I needed.

All I had to do was ask.

When I was finally healed enough that I could hobble around and not have to be stuck in bed anymore, I was ecstatic! My kidney still hurt, but not as bad because I didn't have to lay flat all-day long. I was able to unpack and turn our new place into a home, and I even got to go out in public in my cute maternity clothes. I told myself I was never going to take my freedom and independence for granted again, and I would never take another nap as long as I lived. (Go ahead and laugh, my kids weren't born yet, I had no idea.)

My sweet boy was born via C-section on August 24th, 2011. Just like my entire pregnancy, nothing went as planned during his birth, but all of it was worth it.

All. Of. It.

I look at my son now and silently thank sweet Kenna for helping me keep him safe. If I hadn't been holding her, I may have tried to catch myself, or moved a different way and fell on my stomach; who knows what could have happened. All the issues I had, being stuck in a stuffy room for over two months and the awful pain, they did go away. It did get better, and my baby is now six years old!

Even if your pregnancy is "average," something will likely not go exactly as you planned, but I promise you this: it WILL be worth it. When you hold your baby in your arms for the first time, you'll realize you would do it all over again, and you would do anything for your child.

I clearly remember a specific day when my son was three months old. I was rocking him and thinking back on my pregnancy – that was now mostly a blur. I was so thankful for that time because it brought me my baby, but I was also super grateful it was over. I didn't want to even think about going through pregnancy again. My husband and I talked, and we decided we would begin to think about another baby in three years. God laughed at our plans and a few hours later that same day, I found out I was pregnant again.

But don't worry, that one was worth it all, too.

MY SWEET SURROGACY JOURNEY

BY DANA KAMP

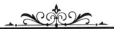

> *"Try not to fear birth. Every single experience is*
> *different, so don't believe yours will be like your cousin's*
> *horrific birth story (or your best friends 'perfect' one).*
> *Go in knowing it will be your unique, amazing,*
> *empowering, and beautiful story."*
> *- 39ish Life*

Giving him to his parents was one of the greatest joys of my life. To watch their tear-streamed faces as he was pulled from my tummy and held in the air, crying and wiggling, red and purple and beautiful, was the most fantastic sight I think I will ever see.

Surrogacy has always been an absolute dream for me. Even as a teenager I thought it would be an incredible experience and wanted to do it "someday." I didn't know when or how it would happen.

Over the years, I shared this dream with my husband, Jeff, and he was always on board. It came up in conversation often as we tried to figure out the timing of adding to our own family and helping build another one.

After our third baby was born, I felt the tug to look into the details of surrogacy. We knew we were going to have a fourth baby at some point, but also knew I would soon cross the age threshold to be considered for a surrogacy. So, we began the process of being put on "the list," and prayed the perfect couple would choose me. In my eyes, "perfect" meant a loving, warm couple eager to be a part of the pregnancy, and who we would become friends with through this awesome experience.

Our first match was with a wonderful couple who we liked right away. We were all ready to proceed until they received fantastic news that a newborn was theirs to adopt if they wanted him. Of course, they jumped at the chance, and we were overjoyed for them!

Jeff and I knew God had a plan for us. And just a few months later, his plan included the happy news that we were expecting our fourth little one! So, my surrogacy file was put on hold for almost two years to allow for my pregnancy and a year of nursing and recovery.

When we were matched again, the couple seemed like a great fit until discussing the vitally important topic of selective reduction. Our attorney's extremely thorough contract covered every possible situation in detail. Both parties had to be on the same page with all of these in order to move forward together. Every surrogate, every person, has the right to decide what she will do in various life situations. For me, I could not agree to put my body through the process of surrogacy, only to end the pregnancy because of a Down syndrome diagnosis or an unwanted multiple pregnancy. This confirmed for me we were not the best match and I asked to be put back on the "Available" list.

Our third match didn't get farther than a strained, uncomfortable Skype chat. I told our attorney it just didn't feel right and to once again put me back on the list.

I knew if I was meant to be a surrogate, and I wholeheartedly believed I was, the perfect match would happen ... at the perfect time.

September 2014 brought the perfect couple, the perfect match, to us. And I knew it within minutes of that first phone call. It seemed so natural and easy to talk to her like we had been friends for years. Then our husbands joined us on a Skype call a few days later, and all four of us just knew.

We flew down to meet them the next month. It was a great visit, finally being able to hang out with them and get excited about what was to come. On that same trip, I had my psychological evaluation and my initial exam with the fertility specialist. The psych exam was mentally tough, but I got through it, and then the physical exam shed light on a small bump in the road. While overall I was in great health, there was a myoma (non-cancerous fibroid) on my uterine wall that needed to be removed before we could proceed. The doctor wanted my body to be as perfect as possible before the embryo transfer.

We scheduled the surgery for January. It was an outpatient procedure done in Miami, and we returned home two days later. We gave my body a few weeks to heal, and then we eagerly jumped into the IVF process.

I had never seen such a precise, intense medication plan. I was given a calendar that spelled out when I should take each pill, apply the numerous patches, and insert each injection over the next several months. I was excited to finally be at this stage of the journey, so the medical part of it didn't bother me at all.

After completing the pre-IVF drug therapy, I had an ultrasound to determine if my body was finally ready. Everything looked great, so the embryo transfer was scheduled for the morning of May 11th. It was painless, but a little awkward, as most appointments in stirrups are. There were two embryos, so we prayed at least one would attach and develop. The biological mommy and Jeff were both in the room with me, and the bio mommy and I were holding hands as the transfer took place. It was serious and clinical but warm and beautiful at the same time.

I stayed on bedrest in the hotel for two days to give my body time to accept the embryos, and then we headed back home. We went back to our regular lives, with a fun little secret only a few friends and family members knew. It would be nine long days before we knew if it was a successful transfer.

The blood test was at 7:30 in the morning, but when the nurses still hadn't called with the results late in the afternoon, I took a pregnancy test at work. I texted a picture of the positive test to the bio mommy, and she called back right away squealing! We couldn't believe it!

The next several weeks were filled with my family's activities (baseball games, field trips, school projects, etc.) and my usual work schedule, with a weekly blood test to make sure my hormone levels were rising. I made two more trips down to Miami in June for appointments with the fertility doctor, and the bio parents traveled up to us in July as we hit the twelve week mark and transferred my prenatal care to my OBGYN. We also found out this miracle baby was a precious little boy! All was moving along wonderfully until the day before Labor Day.

I knew what it was when it happened. My water had broken spontaneously with my third and fourth babies, so I had that exact feeling twice before. But, it was way too early. I was just a few days past nineteen weeks. We rushed to the hospital and were met with solemn faces and sad predictions. We were told there was an enormous chance that I would go into labor or they would need to induce, and he would not survive.

The bio parents drove up that night, and we all agreed we would do anything we could to save this baby. I remember not understanding that there was nothing the doctors could do. I wanted them to stop the leak, to stitch up the tear, to give me some kind of medicine to prevent this from happening. Unfortunately, it was a wait-and-see situation. The small amount of amniotic fluid still around him was sufficient for now, but my risk of infection and the likelihood of contractions beginning worried us all.

I was sent home on strict bed rest and told to return if any signs of labor or a fever appeared. We prayed for my body to hold onto this little guy for just a few more weeks, to get us to that magic "viability" milestone of twenty-four weeks gestation.

Over the next two weeks, we met with a maternal-fetal specialist in hopes of formulating a plan to take us further but were left with tears and diminished hopes that this pregnancy would result in a healthy baby. We decided to transfer to another specialist for a second opinion.

What a difference it made to speak to someone with a positive outlook and a hopeful heart! We knew there was a lot we could not control, but having someone allow us to try something was all we wanted. He agreed to check me into the hospital just shy of twenty-four weeks, where I'd be monitored around the clock until the baby arrived.

Jeff, my parents, my aunt, and a team of babysitters covered all the household duties and childcare for my boys while I was in the hospital. It was so hard to be away from them, but I knew it was necessary to get as far as possible with the pregnancy.

The bio parents came up almost every weekend to visit me and check on the baby. While it wasn't the second trimester we'd envisioned, it did give us more opportunities to grow our relationship and continue fighting as a team.

We celebrated my third son's birthday, Halloween, Jeff's birthday, my birthday, and Thanksgiving while in the hospital, which meant we also celebrated hitting every milestone we were trying to reach. It was remarkable. Ten weeks of daily fetal stress tests, vital checks every four hours, bi-weekly ultrasounds, and periodic blood work led us to a delivery day of December 21st, five days past our ultimate goal of thirty-four weeks.

While I'd imagined a vaginal birth and the doctors handing him to the parents as soon as he arrived, a transverse baby and the unknown condition of his lung development made a C-section the best choice.

Because of our unique circumstances, Jeff and both bio parents were allowed in the operating room, which was also filled with a NICU team, anesthesiologists, nurses, residents, and doctors all ready and anticipating his medical needs. And when that sweet baby was born, and he let out the strongest, most beautiful cry, I don't think there was a dry eye in the room. We did it! We brought this amazing miracle into the world!

And I would do it all over again. That precious little boy, his parents beaming with happiness, the beautiful friendship that was formed. There is nothing more spectacular that could have come from this sweet journey.

WORTH THE WAIT:
THE JOY OF A RAINBOW BABY

JENNIFER BAIROS

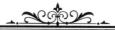

> *"If I got pregnant again, I wouldn't wait three months to tell a few close friends. If I experienced another loss, I would need those people beside me immediately. I would need them to quietly check in with me along the way even if things were going well."*
> *-A Splendid Messy Life*

"Hi, Jennifer. I am just calling to let you know that you are pregnant. Please make an appointment with your family doctor, and we will be in touch soon."

I will never forget this phone call from our fertility clinic. I was sitting upstairs in our den and had been doing something on the computer when the phone rang. We spoke for just a minute; there wasn't much more to say, and then I hung up. The information the nurse gave me felt almost meaningless. After the year I had been through, I had trained myself to be unmoved at the prospect of a potential pregnancy.

Lest I get emotionally attached to the baby.

You see, 365 days before this phone call, and 6 hours from where I actually lived, I was in a hospital recovering from emergency surgery to remove my first miscarriage. I had noticed some bleeding while my husband, Rob, and I were away with friends for the weekend. I knew I was a few weeks pregnant, and Rob and I were both so excited about the idea of becoming parents. We had moved into a new house a few weeks earlier and had even started referring to one of the new rooms as "the nursery." When I saw the blood, we went to the local hospital so I could get checked out. Hours later, my test results indicated that my pregnancy might have been ectopic, and due to the volatile nature of these types of pregnancies, the doctors, rightly, wouldn't let me leave the hospital until I had the necessary surgery to remove the pregnancy.

I was devastated.

I screamed. I cried. I begged them to double check. It had only been a few weeks, but, in my heart, our baby was so real.

Pregnancy loss. Ectopic pregnancy. Miscarriage. Infertility. Grief. These were all terms that had previously sat unused in my vocabulary, and my understanding of them was embarrassingly limited. I believed that these were things "other people" had to deal with. People in the made-for-TV movies. People in other countries. I was young, healthy, and educated. This should not be my story.

And yet, because none of that matters, it was.

Four months later, I had my second miscarriage. It was much less dramatic. Surgery was not required. There was less screaming. There was more crying.

I clung to stories of women who miscarried but went on to have healthy babies. However, in the back of my mind, I feared that I was going to be the one. The one story that wouldn't have a happy ending.

Hope is a funny thing. I don't know about you, but I sometimes find it hard to jump all the way in with hope. So, I had to learn to live with a bit of that scared feeling. What I discovered was that it doesn't mean you're not hopeful. You can feel hope and fear at the same time.

You know that saying, "It takes a village...?" Well, this is where your village comes in. Your partner, your parents, a few close friends. Maybe more. Maybe less. Whoever you know will be there for you. Let them in.

It's hard to talk about sad things, but pregnancy loss is not uncommon. Maybe as even as high as one in four pregnancies end in miscarriage.

That's a lot of sad mamas. Women who need their loved ones to sit with them while they cry. To hold their hands. To make them a cup of tea. To tell them that they are wonderful. To help them pull strength from it all and keep going. To encourage them not to give up hope. Bless our villages.

Fear and hope. That's how I would describe the months that followed. Which brings us back to the fertility clinic and the phone call.

Pregnancy is never the same for someone who has suffered a miscarriage. I don't even really remember being happy the day I found out. I called Rob at work. We didn't say much at the beginning. We both just kind of felt like, "OK. Let's see what happens."

Thankfully, medically, my pregnancy progressed well. At one point my fertility doctor even playfully declared me "boring." He told me to go home and continue being boring.

However, emotionally, my pregnancy left me fraught with conflicted feelings. I yearned to be as happy and excited as I was the first time I ever learned I was pregnant, but it just felt too hard. I couldn't let myself feel joy yet. I was so worried that things could still go wrong.

Early on in my pregnancy, I often felt that this was a kind of "backup baby." I was convinced that my connection with this baby wasn't going to be as strong as it would have been had I never miscarried at all. I was worried that this baby would know he or she wasn't my first choice. I had decided that the baby from my first miscarriage was supposed to be my "real baby," and that I had forever lost my one, real chance at being a mom.

I remember thinking that there was no way I would ever really be able to fully love the child growing inside of me.

This dread kept me from feeling all of the love I wished I could feel.

But the weeks and months passed.

Slowly, tentatively, I began to feel joy with his little kicks. With shopping for his nursery. With watching my belly grow. With hearing his little heartbeat.

Bit by bit, my own heart finally began to believe that this was all going to be okay. We picked out his name: Sebastian. We planned for his baptism. We felt excited.

Remembering those thoughts from early on in my pregnancy still haunts me. I know now that they were a product of the grief I was feeling for those babies that were never to be, but I sometimes still carry guilt when I think of how I used to feel about being pregnant with our son.

From time to time, I wonder about those babies. And even though they were each only a few weeks along, they are still babies to me. I remember them and send warmth and love their way, wherever they are now. I sometimes ask myself what they might have been like. Were they boys or were they girls? Would they have been better sleepers at night? And how would I be different if I hadn't had that year of loss in my life? Would I still have struggled with postpartum depression after Sebastian was born? Would we be more open to trying to have more children?

When these questions come and threaten to spiral within me, all it takes is one of Sebastian's smiles, hugs, or laughs and I know that he was entirely worth this journey. Worth the pain. Worth the tears. Worth the wait. Most importantly, I now know that my fears of being unable to love him fully were completely unfounded.

When I look at our five-year-old, I know in the depths of my heart and my soul that he was the child we were meant to have. I can't imagine him not being here. I can't picture what my life would be like if I hadn't had those miscarriages, and if I had carried a healthy baby to term the first time around. Or the second.

I feel that we are so blessed to be his parents. If I hadn't experienced those two losses, Sebastian wouldn't be here, and I wouldn't get to be his mom. He would never have known the joy of life, and, moreover, we would never have known the joy of him, of who he is, and of the passions and gifts he has to offer.

It's nearly impossible to feel thankful for loss, but for the path that lead me to him, I will be eternally grateful.

So, if any part of my story touches on a part of your story, let me just tell you that it's worth it. It's worth the tears. The fear. The hope when it's hard to hope. When you finally get that little one in your arms, that's when you'll know it was worth the wait.

WHEN ALL YOU CAN DO IS HOPE, PRAY, AND WAIT

WHITNEY HSU

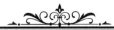

> *"There are some things you won't know until you just know that you know them. Don't worry. Your mama bear instincts will kick in."*
> *- We're Only Hsuman*

Sometimes, a pregnancy doesn't go quite the way you had planned.

When I was pregnant with my third child, I decided that since I was almost thirty, I should have the extra test screening for chromosomal disorders. It's the one that can identify things like Downs syndrome at your first ultrasound around twelve weeks. It's not a required test, but I figured since I was approaching the age where those disorders become more common, I should add it on, even though I did not do the screening with either of my first two children.

The day that I went in for the ultrasound, I was giddy, fantasizing about seeing a little peanut, maybe hands or feet or a little nose. Honestly, you can't see much, but it does become a bit more real to you to see the bouncing jelly bean on that black and white screen. I just knew I'd be able to see a glimpse of a nose or ear that looked familiar. I had a cup of coffee beforehand so I could watch the baby wiggle a little.

Imagine my dismay, then, when the ultrasound tech (the same one I had for my ultrasounds with all of my pregnancies) took a few measurements and got uncharacteristically quiet. She kept moving, trying to get new angles and different measurements. Finally, she spoke slowly and told me she had found something that indicated a "risk" of having an issue. She said that I should have the second screening, which just involved a quick blood draw that day, and I'd get results in a week or so.

Three days later, I was sitting around waiting for the phone call that I was hoping would ease my mind. Of course, my doctor called as I was mid-shower, on a hectic morning, with very little time to process what he was saying. He told me there was a substantial likelihood that the baby, my baby, had Trisomy 18.

If you (like me) don't know anything about it or have never heard of it, here's what the Trisomy 18 foundation says:

Trisomy 18, also known as Edwards syndrome, is a condition which is caused by an error in cell division, known as meiotic disjunction. Trisomy 18 occurs in about 1 out of every 2500 pregnancies in the United States, about 1 in 6000 live births. The numbers of total births increase significantly when stillbirths are factored in that occur in the second and third trimesters of pregnancy.

Unlike Down syndrome, which also is caused by a chromosomal defect, the developmental issues caused by Trisomy 18 are associated with medical complications that are more potentially life-threatening in the early months and years of life. Fifty percent of babies who are carried to term will be stillborn, with baby boys having higher stillbirth rate than baby girls.

Some children will be able to be discharged from the hospital with home nursing support for their families. And although less than ten percent survive to their first birthdays, some children with Trisomy 18 can enjoy many years of life with their families, reaching milestones and being involved with their community. A small number of adults (usually girls) with Trisomy 18 have and are living into their twenties and thirties, although with significant developmental delays that do not allow them to live independently without assisted caregiving.

Cliff's notes: This is bad. High risk of miscarriage. High risk of stillbirth. High risk of infant mortality. Unlikely for my baby to reach his/her childhood years, much less reach the other side of them.

My doctor (who happens to be my hero, based on every interaction with him and his delivery of my other two babies) encouraged me to get a (very expensive but very worth it) blood test that would give us ninety-nine percent accurate results as to whether the baby has Trisomy 18. So there I was, having taken a test that would tell me for almost certain whether or not I should be worried for the next six months, whether or not to even get excited about decorating a nursery and buying a new outfit or two, whether I will have just moments with my sweet child or years. How can a woman possibly be expected to hear this news and do anything but stay in bed all day (several days!) and cry?

As you might expect, I was an emotional wreck. I vacillated between crying and yelling and being silent and praying and pretending I was fine. Just going through my regular motions of feeding the older two children and carrying on conversations in the grocery store required ALL of my energy. I was on an extremely short fuse, bearing the unbearable weight of possible bad news. I carried my phone around with the ringer set to "foghorn" so that I wouldn't miss a message or call from the doctor's office. I jumped at every sound, cried at every thought of what the near future could hold for our family. The very trauma of that waiting has made me extremely sensitive to those who struggle with multiple miscarriages and infertility ever since.

So I'll spare you the waiting and waiting that I went through.

My doctor called late in the afternoon, as I was lying down to nap. When I saw the caller ID, my heart stopped in my chest. I knew it was the moment of truth. My world could either continue turning or be shattered for the foreseeable future. I'd been waiting and waiting for this call, and there I was, unsure if I could even answer it.

But I did, and he (thankfully, blessedly, and PRAISE THE LORD!) told me the test came back negative for Trisomy 18 and a whole host of other chromosomal disorders. He said, "I'm so glad - the baby is normal." THE BABY IS NORMAL! Had anyone ever been so happy to hear about "normal"?! I don't know. But I was ecstatic and overwhelmed and unable to even respond. I just sat and cried on the phone, sniffling and wheezing until my doctor cleared his throat and said he needed to make a few more calls.

The waiting, my friends, is indeed the hardest part. It seemed like an entire lifetime I had waited to hear these results, barely breathing, much less going on with life, until I knew how to proceed, whether I would actually hold this baby. My thoughts were consumed; I didn't stop for a moment to pray for anything else. I just "zombied" my way through a week and a half of life, waiting to hear whether my family would drastically change in a good way or bad.

But my end result isn't always the end result. There are those who receive that horrible call that something is, in fact, very wrong. Those mothers who go in to have the baby, and come home empty-handed. I sit here writing this, three years after I lived it, tears streaming down my face thinking about how it could have gone much, much worse. The waiting was the only hard part for me... it was followed only by joy and life. I know that I'm the lucky one.

Your Growing Family

ALL YOU NEED IS OPTIMISM AND HOT DOGS

BRITON UNDERWOOD

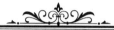

> *"My advice to expectant dads is if she eats cake for breakfast join in on eating. Don't be judgmental!"*
> *- Diana (Punk Rock Papa's Wife)*

I knew my wife, Diana, was pregnant before she did. I'd never seen a woman, or anyone for that matter, go through a pack of hot dogs so quickly. I'm not talking about just the regular eight-pack of hot dogs either. No, I mean the big, family-size, ones you buy if you're hosting people for a barbecue. Knowing my wife hadn't found a sudden passion for competition eating, I gently negotiated a hot dog out of her hand, and replaced it with a pregnancy test.

As I drove to get more hot dogs from the store, reality solemnly hit me in the face. We weren't ready for another baby. Barely of drinking age, we were already young, dumb, parents with our hands full of babies. My wife's first pregnancy gave us beautiful twin boys. Their birth hadn't been easy though. Towards the end, a sudden, dangerous, spike in Diana's blood pressure put her in an emergency delivery and the intensive care unit along with our twins. And now, with that memory fresh in mind, we were looking at all the what-ifs of another pregnancy.

We weren't ready for another child, let alone the possibility of another set of twins. Everything about this second pregnancy felt wrong. It felt irresponsible. We already lived in a small place, with a roommate, and had to share our room with the twins. There was barely enough room for the dog, let alone more children. Our best bet at financially supporting a bigger family would be for me to contact seedy friends from my past and sell my kidneys in a shady back alley.

As wrong as this pregnancy felt, none of the alternatives felt right either. So, we marched fearlessly into the unknown. Our hands filled with hot dogs, and our hearts filled with cautious optimism.

This second pregnancy helped us begin to pull our lives together. We had no choice but to push forward and make this work. After an ultrasound showed us we would only have one this time, we began to look for a bigger place to live. Bolstered by the joy of our firstborns, and this steadily growing excitement of adding to our family, we did what we've always done; we trusted in each other.

Flying on the wings of love, or maybe, more accurately, youthful naivety, we went to doctor's appointment after doctor's appointment. Because of the first pregnancy's complications, Diana fell into the high-risk category. With an amazing team of doctors and technicians assembled around my wife, we moved ever closer to the due date of our new addition.

Somewhere along the way, it just began to feel right. Even when things weren't exactly going our way. We decided this child would be a girl. It wasn't. We found a gorgeous, gigantic, place to live and raise a family. We didn't get it. But, we held on to what we had. Our optimism. Gripping it until our knuckles went white. What choice did we have? Our baby boy was on his way.

Our son would be a Christmas baby. With Diana in the high-risk category, her due date had to be carefully mapped out. He would be delivered on December twenty-sixth, which narrowly crossed the name Christ 2.0 off our list. My push to call him Hot Dog fell on deaf ears. My wife also didn't want to call him; Spanish Jesus, Santa, Nitrate, Dumbledore, or Jacoby.

We decided to go with the name Ezra. I wanted my son to have a unique, strong, name we could never find on a keychain. Having a unique name myself (Briton), I felt the bitterness given to me as I grew up unable to find a custom keychain ultimately built my character and I wanted to pass that on to my son. Ezra Michael Underwood. EMU. We were having an EMU.

As Ezra's due date approached, the pieces to the puzzle fell into place. We found a bigger place. Began to be more fiscally responsible. The pregnancy itself ran smoothly. Ezra utilized all the room his brothers didn't have in the womb. A big boy, measuring around eight pounds, he was happy, healthy, and loved to kick Mommy's bladder. Our months of clinging to optimism resulted in things beginning to come together. Christmas Day quietly came and went. We bundled the twins up, giving them hugs and kisses, and brought them to Grandma's house. We returned to our quiet home to rest for the big day. Laying there that night before, we knew our lives would be changed forever in the morning. Sleep didn't come easily that night. Tossing. Turning. Wondering about how the next day would go.

We got to the hospital too early. A miscommunication with the doctor had us arrive at the hospital a full six hours before the scheduled C-section. I felt bad for my wife. Having to sit there for hours with pre-baby jitters is bad enough, but they made this poor woman starve. When they took us in extra early, they failed to mention they'd immediately limit her to a liquid diet. She had to sit there all morning on an impromptu fast while I ran out to get a breakfast sandwich.

Through her two pregnancies, I've always marveled at the strength my wife possesses. She is fierce. A babe, who rocks motherhood and doesn't let obstacles get in her way. I sat there listening to her poor stomach growl and roar for food, nervous about the impending delivery. She sat binge-watching a t.v show and talking about how good a cheeseburger would be after giving birth. During delivery, she and the doctor talked about what her first post-pregnancy alcoholic drink would be. I sat light-headed on the floor.

Yeah, I passed out and missed the birth. Somewhere between my breakfast sandwich and the five hours of sitting, I hyped the situation up to anxiety attack proportions and lasted about five minutes into delivery until the doctor had to bring me back with smelling salts.

As my wife talked margaritas with her OBGYN, I breathed in and out of a paper bag in a separate room. A part of me felt guilty for missing the birth. The twin's birth had been this whirlwind of rushing from room to room with no time to stop and realize what was happening. It felt like I'd been lying in bed and blinked into fatherhood. With Ezra, I'd had all this build up and preparation. By the time we reached the delivery room, I'd psyched myself out.

While I sat with my bag, my baby boy came into this world kicking and screaming, something he has continued to do in excessive amounts. Diana had her tubes tied right after. According to her, being surrounded by three boys and me was more than enough. She couldn't risk her sanity on trying for a girl.

All the worries surrounding Ezra's birth feel like a lifetime ago. At just three years old, he has this personality, unlike anyone I have ever known. Maybe it's the high levels of nitrate he endured in utero, but the kid is one of the goofiest, clumsiest, kindest people I have ever met. His smile, a possible byproduct of the nine months we spent pushing forward with positivity in spite of everything feeling hopeless at times, is contagious.

A lot of worries surrounded Ezra's arrival, but we never once didn't want him. When he came, and we got to hold him for the first time, everything finally felt right. My baby boy, little Ezra Michael Underwood. Emu, as we affectionately call him.

He makes our family whole.

And, boy, does that child love hot dogs.

FIRST COMES LOVE THEN COMES BABY

TIFFANY O'CONNOR

"Women have a tendency to rely on the females in their own family when they are pregnant. If your partner is close to his mother make an effort to include her... even if you don't get along. Let her plan the baby shower, ask her for advice about breastfeeding, and make sure she knows what is going on with her growing grandchild. Your partner will appreciate you for it"
– James (Tiffany's Husband #Lifewithboys)

You fell in love, and one thing leads to another, and now you are pregnant. You are probably wondering how pregnancy and parenthood are going to change your romantic relationship. Everyone has heard the jokes about how having kids kills your sex life...it doesn't have to. Raising a family together can bring you closer if you remember to put your partner first. He was there before you got pregnant and with a lot of hard work and a little luck he will still be there after your kids have grown up and have all moved out of the house.

It's no secret that the woman has to carry the majority of the burden of pregnancy. However, while you are pregnant, there are several ways to involve your partner and deepen your bond. This is also the last time that it will be just the two of you, so it's important not to get so wrapped up in the baby that is coming that you forget to focus on each other.

Pregnancy Sex

With my first pregnancy, my OBGYN was the same doctor who delivered my husband, and possibly Moses, and probably a few dinosaurs. So it was almost impossible at twenty-one to bring myself to discuss sex with my extremely elderly male doctor. All of the popular pregnancy books told me that it was ok, but it made us nervous, and we mostly avoided it… which was really hard because we were used to having sex almost daily. The lack of physical intimacy mixed with the financial burden of an unplanned pregnancy while we were still very young left us feeling distant and emotionally strained.

With my second pregnancy, we got a new female OBGYN with five of her own children and a habit of forcing us to ask questions and open up to her before she would allow us to leave her office. One of my husband's biggest concerns was whether or not we could still have sex while I was pregnant, because the idea of another year without sex was not something he wanted to endure. My doctor didn't just assure him that in most pregnancies sex was ok and wouldn't hurt the baby, she also offered suggestions.

That's right. As if having her staring at my vagina all the time wasn't awkward enough she started giving us in-depth pregnancy sex advice.

She told us that spooning or lying on the bed with him standing between my legs would be the easiest positions once my belly started to grow. She explained that oral sex for me could be dangerous because air blown into my vagina could cause a blood clot but that she highly recommended oral sex for him when I didn't want to be touched down there (which is actually good period sex advice too). She explained that pregnancy sex in the second trimester might actually feel a lot better than normal and that was because of increased blood flow to the pelvis, increased vaginal lubrication, and heightened sensitivity of the nipples and to just enjoy that time as much as possible. She was right by the way…second-semester pregnancy sex is AWESOME!!

She also suggested 'thigh sex' for the third trimester. Go ahead Google it. I'll wait…It's totally a thing. A thing my husband and I could never figure out. However, we still randomly bring it up and laugh just as hard as we did the first time she mentioned it. It's become one of those weird jokes between us that every married couple has.

Intimacy

I know we already talked about sex, but there are other forms of intimacy that are just as important when you are pregnant. It's a time when you really have to rely on the closeness and friendship that you have. You have to drop all of your boundaries once you are pregnant because you have to be able to rely on each other from now on in ways you never have before. You're becoming a team. A team that is going to have to raise an entire person together. A team that will have to be solid when that cute newborn turns 13 and wants to play you against each other to get what he wants. Discuss EVERYTHING. Not just your fears and your dreams but also the small things like what you want family holidays to look like with a child (should you plan cute family themed Halloween costumes and do either of you really want to drive to six different Thanksgiving dinners to make every family member happy?) or which pets your partner is not allowed to bring home no matter how much your offspring beg. (For me it's a cat... cats are my pet hard limit)

If you have never farted or pooped in front of your partner. Let that crap go...literally. You are going to frequently be gassy during the next nine months and there is nothing worse than trying to lift your huge whale baby body off the couch to go fart in the other room sixteen times while watching a movie and honestly if you give vaginal birth you are probably going to crap on the delivery table, and you most likely don't want that to be the first time your partner realizes that you do in fact poop. Plus, there will be other somewhat embarrassing situations that will arise when you are pregnant. You will get to the point where you can no longer see your toes, which will also mean you can no longer shave your legs and lady parts by yourself. So unless you want to show up to the hospital with Chewbacca legs and a full bush (unless that's already your thing), you are going to have to ask your partner to do it for you. I can't even describe the level of intimacy it takes to allow someone else to use a razor near your fragile body parts.

Talking about embarrassing situations. There will be things that happen while you are pregnant that you will need your significant other for. I once drove over a pothole in my company vehicle when I was eight months pregnant and peed myself. My husband had to bring me a change of clothes and help me steam clean the driver's side seat because my boss needed the car in an hour and I didn't want to have to tell my boss that I peed all over the seat of the car. I also once peed myself and thought it was my water breaking. My husband took off of work to rush me to the hospital just to have the ER doctor inform us that my underwear was covered in urine and not amniotic fluid. He didn't laugh at me or get angry...he just got me cookies and cream ice cream on the way home and rubbed my back while I sobbed on the couch that night...half from embarrassment and half because I really wanted that kid out of me and I was pissed that I was still pregnant. I honestly don't think I could have cried like that or eaten a whole carton of ice cream in front of anyone but him.

Getting Ready For the Baby

When I found out I was pregnant with our first child, I rushed out to the library and borrowed all of the popular pregnancy books. I didn't ask my husband if he wanted to read them. I just assumed that he wouldn't. To be honest, I wasn't even that great at reading them. The medical stuff overwhelmed me, and I was so scared of labor that I couldn't bring myself to read about it. Instead, I opted for watching those pregnancy shows that make you scared that every time the baby hiccups or you get a cramp that you have some rare disease that is going to kill you or the baby...because that was obviously better than reading the medical jargon in the pregnancy books. Every time that I would tell him about my latest symptom that obviously pointed towards impending doom, he would tell me exactly what was going on, and it would ease my fears.

I was never sure how he knew and assumed it was something he picked up when his older sisters were pregnant. Until the day I opened the bathroom door to find him sitting on the toilet reading one of those pregnancy books that I was too scared to read. I learned that he had read EVERY single one of them. (For the libraries sake I am hoping he didn't read them all on the toilet) He was afraid of losing the baby or me, and the information in the books made him feel better when I was freaking out and helped him to be able to reassure me (and himself) that everything was going to be ok.

There were other things he did with me to get ready for our sons to be born when I was pregnant. He took the Lamaze class with me during our first pregnancy. We both got out of watching those graphic videos second time around…Yay for planned C-sections! He registered for my baby showers with me, and I resisted the urge to unregister for the PlayStation or super expensive fishing pole that he was sure our newborn baby would need. I kind of just hoped that his Aunts would realize that he scanned those items and not me. With our second son, I even let him pick out the baby bag because I realized that he was probably pretty embarrassed carrying around the bright baby blue one with elephants on it when our oldest was little and honestly I really liked the sleek black one that he picked out.

We gave in to my cravings together. Sympathy weight happens, and it happens because when you send him to get tacos in the middle of the night, he is going to eat some too. Don't worry he will lose all of his by giving up soda and bread for a week and it will take you nine years to lose yours (Ok…maybe that is just me). My husband painted both of our son's rooms while we were preparing for their arrivals (apparently paint fumes are not good for pregnant ladies) and he built the cribs which were both second hand, so they didn't come with directions and probably had missing parts. We went to every doctor's appointment together, and he asked the questions that I was afraid to ask. During our last ultrasound appointment he even asked the ultrasound tech to show him and our oldest son where the bathroom was (he thought he was being slick, but I know he knew where the bathroom was) so I could shed a few tears without an audience in disappointment after learning that our second (and last) child was going to be another boy.

We picked our children's names together. Our first son was easy because we knew what we were going to name him before he was even conceived. Cannon was named after a kid I nannied that we were both fond of. Plus Cannon O'Connor seemed like it would be a kick-ass football player name and now that he is his junior highs quarterback having the name Cannon is pretty fitting. Naming our second son was more of a challenge. At one point the argument got so heated that I threw a lamp…I blame pregnancy hormones. My husband's top three choices were Lucas, Eugene, and Randy.

I couldn't stand the thought of our son being called 'Luke the Puke' or myself embarrassing my child by screaming 'Wandy' in front of his friends because even after years of speech therapy my R's still occasionally come out as W's when I am frustrated or angry.

He really wanted to give our second child a name with family significance, so he consulted several different baby name books until he found Cullin. His mother's maiden name was Cullinane and Cullin seemed to fit with Cannon perfectly. Cullin meant bear cub in Irish and Cannon meant wolf cub, and they seemed like the perfect names for the O'Connor brothers. If I hadn't let him take the lead picking our son's name instead of being the only Cullin in his class, he would have most likely been one of the five Aiden's or Jackson's because I would have gone with something entirely too trendy.

Pregnancy isn't easy. To be honest, I am one of those people who hated it. But every swollen ankle and Braxton Hicks contraction was worth it the very moment I saw the love of my life holding the child that we made together. I have to admit there are still moments that I will drop back behind my husband and sons while we are walking as a family so I can take in the amazing view of my boys walking next to their father talking to him about life. When we have problems or arguments and things get tough (because EVERY marriage gets tough) I remember that my husband is my best friend and that he loves me so much that he could still look at me puffy eyed from crying about peeing myself while wolfing down an entire carton of ice cream and tell me that I was beautiful…and ladies when you find that kind of love you hold on to it with both hands.

So put this book down (just for tonight, you are going to want to read the rest of it), give your partner a kiss, and make your own memories that will get you through the rough days.

HOW STRANGE: THE SECOND BABY IS DIFFERENT THAN THE FIRST

ABIGAIL HAWK

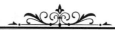

> *"Kegels now, or forever be unable to hold your pee."*
> *-Abigail Hawk*

I wake with a start at 2 am and think, how strange. Not because of the ungodly hour, as 2 am is as constant a bedfellow as my husband and the cat, but because the sheets are soaked. I have gestational diabetes; had I wet myself? It was within the realm of possibility. But no; everything smells sweet, not sour. And, upon investigation, I discover the dam has sprung a leak; I am in fact leaking amniotic fluid. Five weeks early.

This isn't altogether unexpected. My hospital bag has been packed for several weeks now. After all, your brother came five weeks early too, after previous (and thankfully thwarted) entrances at 25 weeks and 32. After all, this second pregnancy has not been so easy on me. Diabetes, edema, insomnia, sciatica, the shots of progesterone, and indigestion. We wake the neighbor to stay with your brother. I kiss him goodbye, shove my shattered heart aside, feel a stubborn tear squeeze out uninvited. He will no longer be my one and only. How strange.

We drive. Me, containing my leak with a super pad. Me, wearing my buffalo plaid wrap coat. It has a big red riding hood, and it ties above my belly. It isn't very warm, but it perfectly buffers my wolverine hot flashes from the winter bite, so it serves me well. Hood up and wolf away, I waddle, penguin-like, through the ER bay, calmly saying, "My water has broken." The security guard wears a neon yellow watch. It stands out in sharp contrast against the nondescript color of his uniform. It reads a touch after

3. I stand before the elevator doors, unable to recall the floor I need. Push 11, he says. I give him a Mona Lisa smile.

In the elevator, I realize I am officially in labor. How strange. I don't feel like I'm in labor. I feel serene. I screamed like a banshee with your brother. So much fear and indecision over pain management and physical limits. My contractions were a contrast of purpose and pain, pretzel-ing me into one of those medieval torture devices that quarters its victims in opposing directions. The seas were violent and wretched. I was Dr. Jekyll and Mr. Hyde. But. All is quiet with you. The elevator beeps softly as I journey upward, calm seas and steady horizon. How strange.

More beeps now. I watch you breathe. Tiny hat and tiny swaddle encompass you snugly, where, mere moments ago, that was my job. We were strangers sharing space. Blood strangers spooning, you in my womb, a letter neatly tucked in my envelope, a bunny in my burrow. And now, here you are, sprawled before me, a tiny stranger who I've somehow known my whole life. We've breastfed a couple of times now, your little mouth rooting for my nipple, my jaw gritted with determination, grimacing every time you succeed. It hurts so much. I remember this with your brother. I remember being chapped and raw and bloody and calloused and hard. But my will was harder, and I persevered. I silently promise I will with you, too.

I cannot feel my legs. The epidural failed, fruitless, and I felt everything for a seeming eternity, but then it kicked in hot and heavy, and I felt nothing but frustration. I wanted to be present, mentally and physically, to feel the pressure, the way I felt your brother, the way I knew the moment his head emerged, one shoulder, then the other... but instead my legs were held spread eagle, and I pushed you here while my lower half lay prostrate and sleeping. The only indication I had that I was working was the clutching of my better half's hand, warm and steady, and the deep breaths I craved but couldn't quite complete. These efforts reassured me, but still, I watched your arrival from above, laboring paralytically. How strange.

We drive. With your brother, I held my organs in place and screamed in pain the whole car ride home, terrified the smallest jerk would snap his neck or eject him. But I make no such screams now. I make phone calls, instead, to your brother's school, to my job, to the curious and congratulatory. I wrap my abdomen tightly, leaving just enough space to inspire. I efficiently filter others' elation, funneling the feelings to their aortic bedchambers; like Mary, I keep these things. I ponder them in my heart. But my heart burns. It threatens to burst from its ribbed barrier, for I am so in love with you, you see. It is this instantaneous thing. How strange.

With your brother, I did not feel love-at-first-sight imprinting of souls. My devotion burned steadily. With you, it is hungry, ferocious and wild, the growing pains an all-consuming conflagration. I seek to feed it, to sew you to me. But you won't latch. I can't satisfy you. You eat as if it bores you, casually grazing, luxuriating. You mock my battle with insomnia as if you instinctively grasp that sleep is an elusive mate but 2 am is friendly. I find myself defeated; my heat snuffed out.

I recant my silent promise to nurse you, and I pump instead. You are now "bottle-fed." My companions become a hard kitchen chair and a pink pumping bra and a black granite counter and a crushing sense of guilt. Your father holds you shirtless, skin to skin, bonding you to him, and I sit with my feet on the cold tile floor. I connect with a machine that evicts my milk and squishes my nipples with a relentless errr eeee errr eeee errr eeee, its reverie only broken by the thrum of the aquarium filter. I am lonely. The cold creeps up like the serpent of Eden, beckoning me to slip under, calling me to darkness. Sometimes, I eat his dark fruit. Sometimes, I think it would be so easy. Sometimes, I lose myself in nausea and cellulite and ovarian torsion and sleepless nights and blood sugar spikes. I overflow with self-loathing. Water pools in my ankles, feeding the root systems of purple trees. Or maybe they are vein tributaries, small streams winding their way to the crook of my knee. My hair is a field of dry wheat. With your brother, it fell out and returned lush and soft, new growth, a new season. But it's brittle now, and it won't fall out. It just hangs there like chaff, like ash spaghetti. The night's negative spaces hang the moon.

But mornings come, and coffee helps. A fresh pot brews, the beans bitter and strong. I pour in some almond milk and contemplate the fake coral in the aquarium. The tank needs cleaning; the dog needs to be fed; your brother's lunch needs packing. Tasks beg my attention. But I pause and take stock of me taking up space. The landscape of my corporeal form is new. My hips have shifted; there are new dimples, new hills and handles with which I retain water and hold you. New pale stretch marks have broken ground as if some sharp-nailed witch drew spells down my buttocks with white chalk, tattooing protective lines of maternal instinct into my skin. Gravity has pulled my breasts further down like small mountains after a mudslide. My areolas bend in awkward angles, broken tilt-a-whirls. They still spit milk sometimes, as if they seek your lips. How strange.

The sky is ablaze with radiant color; a laser beam of sunlight streams through the kitchen window, temporarily blinding me, and it reminds me: the soul that breaks open contains the whole universe. It is there in the golden ratio swirl of your hair and the logarithmic spiral of your fingerprints. There are Fibonacci-sequenced galaxies in your eyes and constellation freckles scattered across your nose, and your fingernails are crescent moons, and your skin is made of star stuff. And I tell myself I'll soon shave with ease. I'll soon sleep for 5 hours straight. I'll soon see you smile, new teeth breaking forth like crocus shoots in spring. I tell myself it's okay to be sad. Picasso painted miracles during his Blue Period. And I tell myself it's okay to be tired. God rested on the seventh day. I tell myself it's okay.

GENDER DISAPPOINTMENT: BONDING WITH BABY THE SECOND TIME AROUND

AARONICA COLE

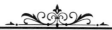

> *"It's ok to not love being pregnant. You see all these people running half marathons while looking like goddesses and that's not everyone pregnant. And it's ok if that's not you."*
> *- The Crunchy Mommy*

I feel like an ungrateful mother every time I think and share my pregnancy experience with my second child affectionately known as ABC. My first pregnancy was hard. I puked four times daily from the time I was eight weeks pregnant until my oldest was one-month-old. It was awful. But I loved being pregnant with her. The minute I felt her move in my belly my purpose in the world was restored. She was my unplanned blessing that I nurtured alone and poured into.

Shortly after my husband and I got engaged, we found out that we were pregnant. Let me tell you this, no matter how many Google results tell you that it takes at least three months to get pregnant after the Mirena is removed DO NOT LISTEN! We had the Mirena removed in October, and by November ABC was hanging out in my belly. The early symptoms were similar: I was insanely tired, overly emotional, and my boobs hurt--this symptom was new for me. I took about five tests before one finally came back positive.

We were pregnant.

I was not as excited as I should have been.

It's crazy because I really should have been over the moon. We had "planned" for this baby. But I wasn't exactly ready to be pregnant just yet.

Though we knew we wanted to get pregnant relatively soon, I just hadn't expected it to be so fast, and that threw me for a loop. That and then finding out ABC was a she.

I just knew she was a boy. We had only discussed boy names. When I was fourteen weeks, we went to see if we would be able to find out the gender of my budding baby. The ultrasound tech excitedly typed out "IT'S A GIRL!!!" on the screen, and my heart dropped.

Wrong.

She had to be wrong, right? It felt like I was pregnant with a boy. The energy was so different this time that I knew she was wrong. I told her we would be back in two weeks so that we could see things more clearly. And at sixteen weeks she gave the final answer: we were having another girl. I was NOT happy. In my disappointment, I didn't even ask if she had all her fingers and little toes. I was too caught up in my hormonal pity party to check on the health of my baby. Looking back on this experience now, I'm pretty disappointed in myself.

Because ABC was a girl and not the boy that I had wanted, I was having a tough time bonding. I'd felt her move, and I didn't fall in love the way that I did when my oldest moved. I almost resented her. But then at twenty-two weeks, I got sick. I was throwing up a lot which wasn't normal for this pregnancy. Outside of the throwing up, my entire body hurt and felt weak. This was a Sunday. I stayed in bed all day and Monday I felt a little better. I called out from work and decided to get some things done around the house that I wasn't able to the day before. As I was out grocery shopping, I began to feel pains that were like contractions. I ignored the pain as I talked to my mom until I was in so much pain I couldn't ignore them anymore. She told me to go to my doctor right away and not bother to call first.

She stayed on the phone with me as I drove to my doctor barely able to walk in. They told me that I was dehydrated which was causing the contractions. I sat down and drank some water which did nothing, so I drove myself to their location that was close to the hospital. My husband met me there--I was hobbling out in tears because no one in the office bothered to see the pain that I was in. I was headed to the hospital.

I was checked in right away, and my contractions were coming faster and faster. I was in early labor. They tried to find a vein to put an IV in, but all my veins were flat because of the dehydration. They managed to draw blood and get an IV into my hand which is how they found out that my white blood count was quadruple what it should have been. I was sent to get an ultrasound immediately because they couldn't tell if there was an infection around the baby or if it was just in my body. If it was around the baby, they would have to take her, and she wouldn't survive.

There was a chance my baby wouldn't survive.

I was devastated as they wheeled me down to the ultrasound tech. I don't know if I've ever prayed as hard as I did in those thirty minutes. The ultrasound took about five minutes before he showed me my baby in my belly sucking her thumb as the contractions came. She was trying to soothe herself, and I fell in love. He cleared us, and I wanted to hug him but, well, IV's in the hand made that difficult.

As they rolled me back to my room, my husband and mom came down the hall, and it was the first time I smiled as I told them WE were ok. My girl and I would be fine. We stayed in the hospital a total of three days and had five bags of IV over those days. I missed being home with my husband and eldest daughter, but I really enjoyed the time that I had with the baby in my belly. I started talking to her and singing to her. I called her by her name and prayed all the prayers of thanks.

When my hospital stay was over, my mom came to pick me up. We enjoyed lunch and some quality thrifting together before we headed back to my house. I was my mom's third pregnancy, and I'm sure that our bond developed differently since I was her rainbow baby but having her there was also the reminder that I needed of what motherhood is. Motherhood is showing up for your children even when you live six hours away, and you might not be on the best terms. It's laughing together, fighting, but loving through it all.

I've been lucky that I've had all healthy babies. While I will never tell another mother how to feel about the baby inside of her what I will say is this: just like each baby is different, so is each pregnancy and each bond with that baby. For some moms, you fall in love the instant you find out and that's beautiful. For others, it takes time, and that's ok. The important thing is that you love hard and you don't give up on them. Plus, let's be real: babies are easy to love so get that foundation down! When they become toddlers, it'll test that bond ha!

TICKLED PINK

KARSSON HEVIA

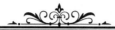

> *"I've never felt more in love or insane. Remember
> in motherhood, when you think you can't take
> it anymore, the tides change and things get easier.
> And wine. There's always wine."*
> ~ *Too Many Open Tabs*

Early in our relationship, my now husband and I would talk at length about kids; and not if we wanted them, but rather, how soon. We'd consider the typical talking points of financial security, our status in the corporate world, and our long-term aspirations as individuals and as a couple. I remember so clearly, my mom bestowing a wise piece of advice to me, which was, 'if you wait until you're ready to have kids, you'll never have them.' How true a statement that is! When the right time came for us to start growing our family, I'd always envisioned having a daughter, no matter what. It just seemed like ponytails, barrettes, Barbies and tutus were somehow part and parcel to my image of motherhood. Coming from a fairly female-dominated household growing up, it was just the natural scene: life was spent quietly playing with coloring books, making bracelets and creating dance recitals in the basement —there were no wrestling matches, race tracks or fart jokes.

Then I became pregnant with my first child. A beautiful baby boy with dimples for days and a determined spirit that would rival some of the greatest leaders. Adapting to a life of raising a boy was different. He was, quite simply, wired differently from me. His motivations, aspirations and topics of interest were ones that didn't come instinctively to me. I had to learn to love to watch construction sites day-after-day, play Matchbox cars and watch cartoons with superheroes...and I did. I evolved into the quintessential 'boy mom' almost overnight, embracing his love for all things that made him happy, and in turn, me too.

Three years later, I found myself learning that once again, we'd be delving even deeper into the boy world, with yet another little dude on the way. Of course, my husband was elated, immediately envisioning our boys as dominating half the outfield, which pleased him to no end. We'd only ever discussed having two, my knee-jerk reaction of more than that made my anxiety immediately elevated. *"I don't want to be outnumbered by my kids"*, I'd think to myself, *"when it's not one-on-one anymore, that when anarchy comes into play — we need to maintain the upper hand."* And it's true; three kids is a big responsibility and huge lifestyle change. Now you require a bigger car, a bigger house, a bigger table. Everything becomes a much larger scale.

We welcomed our new addition to our family joyfully, and our new little bundle fit the textbook personality of a classic second-born. He entered the world laidback. He was easygoing, flexible, accommodating, and had an abundance of light-hearted zest for life. It was a refreshing contrast to that of our older son who at three, believed he knew mostly everything there was to know about the world already and whose spirit was always serious and unwavering. Watching the two of them blossom into best friends and create a harmonious balance within our world, has been nothing short of incredible to watch. Hudson takes some of Hawkins go-with-the-flow ideology and Hawk gleans some of Hudson's steadfast determination and cerebral tenacity.

All this said, I still felt like my picture wasn't entirely complete, my story unfinished. And while my original depiction of what motherhood would look like for me has changed significantly over the course of seven years, I couldn't help but shake the feeling that I just felt unfinished. So, cue the long talks and midnight deliberations over what to do. Ironically, when Hawkins was only two months old, my husband was rearing to go again and wanted to have another. Now, ask any mother whose child is two months if their ready to do it all over again, and unequivocally, the answer is always 'no!' So, we'd tabled the conversation until three years later, and my husband found himself happy with our family of four and didn't want to upset the applecart. I get it; we were in a good groove. Everyone was happy and healthy and SLEEPING! But, I knew our journey didn't end there. So, several months and many pregnancy tests later, I got the double pink line and couldn't be more excited…and terrified… but mostly excited.

This time around, instead of prematurely picking out names and thinking of what this baby was, I lead with the fact that more than likely it was another boy, and I couldn't wait to find out what intrinsic personality lay ahead.

Being that I would be thirty-five by the time of delivery, the medical community preemptively stamped me with the tag of 'Advanced Maternal Age' (sounds lovely, doesn't it?), and concluded that despite my healthy lifestyle and history of healthy pregnancies, I was to take several tests earlier in the pregnancy to rule out any abnormalities. Fine. I conceded and figured that at least then I'd be able to start planning earlier for my third little dude. I took the blood test on a Wednesday and was told to expect the results in seven to ten days. I didn't. I heard back that following Monday, and to say that I was shocked to hear from my midwife that soon, is the gravest understatement.

I'll never forget the call. I saw her number show up on the caller id on my phone and immediately my heart started to race with anticipation. She promptly explained she'd gotten back my results and asked if I wanted to hear them. Now, anyone who knows me knows that I'm about as impatient as they come, and so the idea of not choosing to hear the results is as crazy to me as not taking a handout of a free diamond ring. Get my point? So, I immediately assured her that yes, I did, in fact, want to find out the results, but needed to breathe for just a minute to catch up with my heart rate, which now felt like a marching band booming in my chest. She first began with the fact that I could thankfully be rest assured that my genetic results came back with a negative result for all chromosomal abnormalities. Whew! As if pregnancy isn't challenging enough with a host of other issues, we have to anguish over issues with the baby for months before knowing — it's excruciating. So I, of course, was over the moon with learning the clean bill of health of our little one, but now came time to learn the gender. I started by saying, "As you know, we have two little guys already, and so we'd be happy…" and that's when she cut me off and immediately exclaimed, "Karsson, you're having a GIRL!" Everything after that moment truly seemed to happen in slow motion. My voice seemed foreign and somewhat automated, a disbelieving chant of 'no way, no, omg you're serious?' Kept coming from my mouth like a skipping record on a record player. My ears and hands seemed to go numb, as if my body were weightless, floating. After a couple of minutes of my bizarre chant, she must have recognized my state of shock and told me that she was so happy for us and that I should call my husband with the news. MY HUSBAND! YES! Omg, I had to tell my husband, whom also secretly was rooting for a girl, but didn't want to add any fuel to my already smoldering fire.

I called him at work, no answer. I called him on his cell, no answer. I called him again on his cell and again, no answer. I then texted him with the message of 'URGENT- call me!' — To which he did immediately. After finding out everything was ok, he asked if he could call me back, he was in meeting in the boardroom with seven people staring back at him. I, of course, in my irrational mindset, told him absolutely not, and that I'd found out. Found out what? He'd retorted. SERIOUSLY?!?!? "I found out we're having a girl!' Through many tears of joy and utter disbelief, we reveled in our new exciting news as parents, finally able to allow ourselves the chance of 'trying on' what it would be like to parent a baby girl.

After telling the boys that they're going to be big and even bigger brothers to a baby sister, they both were extremely excited, and lots of precious questions immediately ensued. It was a treasured moment I'll never forget in my entire life and one with which I've since revisited in my head so many times thereafter. I'm in disbelief at the opportunity to parent both boys, and a girl— a dream that I've always thought would never be realized. One thing I know for sure is that even though I've spent the last seven years of motherhood loving, caring for, and refining my boy mom skills, I can't wait for the journey ahead raising my baby girl, and let's be honest, I'm pretty excited to reacquaint myself with Barbies.

Tales From The Labor Room

HOW PRETERM LABOR CHANGED MY LIFE

ANDREA MULLENMEISTER

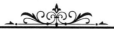

> *"It's always possible to find a silver lining. The harder*
> *it is to find, the brighter it will shine."*
> *-An Early Start*

I'd never known a preemie baby before my son was born. Preterm birth was something abstract, something that only happened to other people. Mainly people who were irresponsible, careless, and unhealthy. It was something that could be prevented if only the mother had taken better care of herself during her pregnancy.

The only picture I had ever seen of a preemie was an Anne Geddes photo of a tiny baby dwarfed by her father's hands. And that baby looked so cute and healthy!

What was the big deal? Weren't preemies just miniature versions of healthy, full-term kids?

So, when I went into preterm labor seventeen weeks before my due date, honestly, I wasn't scared. I guess it's true: ignorance is bliss.

I distinctly remember the split second I went from thinking "this is going to be ok" to terrified. I saw the look on the doctor's face. I remember thinking...holy shit – if she's this scared, then I should be, too!

And then the whirlwind started.

People descended like a swarm of bees to prepare me for a helicopter flight to a larger hospital. A searing pain spread through my arm as a nurse stung me with a steroid shot to strengthen my baby's lungs. I reached out for my husband Steve's hand, but he was lost among the paramedics, nurses, and doctors.

They started a magnesium drip to slow my contractions. My blood turned to liquid lava the second the medicine hit my bloodstream. Fire pulsed through my veins with a ferocity that took my breath away. A nurse slipped an oxygen mask over my face. Paramedics heaved me to a transport board and secured me with six restraints as we rushed outside.

I heard the helicopter before I saw it. The thumping sound vibrated into my bones. Hot afternoon sun blinded me as they loaded me into the roaring machine. I yelled for my husband. For anyone, really. But it was too loud; everyone was busy trying to save the life of my unborn baby.

I was alone.

The paramedic put earphones on my head. I could hear him! He told me he would take care of me. I looked into his kind, blue eyes and said: "I'm afraid of heights." Another contraction ravaged my body as the helicopter rose into the sky. My heart rate rose too from the adrenaline and medicine. I wanted to curl up into a ball, but the restraints kept me from moving.

The paramedic saw on the monitor that another contraction was starting. He took my hands and soothed "I'll ride it out with you." As the contraction started, I yelled "SHIT!" over and over again. Pretty soon, the paramedic was yelling it, too. And then the pilot joined in. We were all yelling swear words at the top of our lungs, and it made me laugh. It was a terrified, panic-y laugh, but it was a laugh all the same. I wondered if anyone else was listening over the radio.

The twenty-five-minute flight felt like twenty-five years.

When we landed, a new team of people rushed me through the hospital doors. I remember looking up at the EMTs who were running down the hall with me, and I curled my body around the bed rail as tight as I could, hoping that would keep the baby in longer. And, at that moment, I knew that prematurity was about to change my life.

The doctor told me to push, I screamed from the depths of my soul "No – I will not have this baby today!"

But my water broke, and my baby came tumbling out, bruised and battered and not breathing. "It's too small." I cried. I tried to get up so I could go to my baby, but the nurse pushed me back onto the bed.

Then I heard one tiny cry - he was alive!

When the nurse handed me the consent form, I had no idea what I was signing. I had no idea the life of my newborn baby was literally in my hands. At that moment, I did not know that babies born too soon are babies who are often born sick. They spend days, months, even years in Intensive Care Units. They have reduced chances of survival; the earlier they are born, the lower those chances are. What I did know was that I was willing to give my baby every chance he needed to grow into a kind, funny, and smart human being. I believed in him. And I signed the paper permitting to use "all means necessary" to keep him alive.

My son was whisked away to the neonatal intensive care unit (NICU) before we decided on his name. My empty arms ached with the magnitude of what had happened. I had just delivered my baby, but I didn't feel like his mother. A mother was supposed to be happy. A mother was supposed to know what her baby looked like. A mother was supposed to whisper "welcome, little one" and not wail as her baby vanished out the door before she could hold him.

Nothing had gone according to plan.

My husband wheeled me to my son's incubator four hours later. I didn't know if my son would live or not, but I made a conscious decision to love him anyway. Everything else was apparently out of my hands.

I peered into the nest of tubes and wires and saw my baby kicking and flailing. He was fighting. At that moment, I knew I would fight, too. There was no doubt left in my heart.

I was Jaxson's mother.

Now, prematurity is real.

Not a day goes by that I do not think about prematurity and how it changed our lives. Now I know that it can happen to anyone. Now I know that it can happen even when a mother takes excellent care of herself during pregnancy. Now I know that babies born too soon often fight the good fight only to earn their angel wings much too early.

Now I also know that babies born too soon can overcome all odds and do more than survive.

It's been five years since Jaxson's whirlwind arrival. Honestly, I have mostly healed from the trauma of his birth. I no longer panic when I hear a helicopter. I'm not worried I will break his bones or rip his skin when I hold him. I have almost forgotten the way my stomach dropped when his neonatologist told me he had a four percent chance of healthy survival.

The intenseness of having a micro-preemie in the NICU has faded. But it's not gone. No, not at all. It's just morphed into regular life. Instead of surviving prematurity, we're living prematurity. Autism, ADHD, asthma and acute respiratory failure, developmental delay. Therapies, appointments, specialists. Medicaid, waivers, insurance.

It's just how we roll. Our life now can't be separated from our life then.

I've learned to be grateful for healthy days, for uneventful hospital stays, and for getting caught up on paperwork. I've learned to advocate for my boy at school and at the doctor's office and hospital to make sure he's getting what he needs.

I've learned how to be the best possible mom to Jaxson. He is happy. He's funny and kind and curious.

When he giggles and leans in for a hug, I am reminded how lucky I am. He's here.

MY LAST PREGNANCY: AN INDUCTION STORY

KAREN JOHNSON

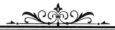

> *"Own this time because it's yours. Husband's giant sweatshirt comfy? WEAR IT. Want to rock cute maternity wear and take professional photos? DO IT. Because once that little bugger comes out, it's game on."*
> *- The 21ˢᵗ Century SAHM*

It was late February, five years ago. I was very pregnant with my third child. Like VERY. PREGNANT. My other two kids had been tanks of babies at birth (over nine pounds), and this little man showed every sign of following in his sister and brother's footsteps. I was due in a few days. Nearing the end of the tunnel. Seeing the light. Grandma and Grandpa were on standby, waiting for the call to watch our four and two-year-old. The hospital bag was packed with the essentials—comfy pants and slippers. (I knew by the third kid just what I needed.) And the car seat was ready to roll.

And then a blizzard hit. Now, depending on where you live, a snowstorm is either catastrophic or like a regular Tuesday. In Kansas, it can go either way. We aren't northern Minnesota, but we aren't southern California either. For Kansas, though, this storm was a biggie. The plows were overwhelmed and working around the clock to clear main roads, so our happy little cul-de-sac was neglected on day one. Then came day two. Still snowed in. Still no school for the kids. Still no work for the husband. And still no ability to leave the house.

We were in full panic mode, knowing that it was unlikely we could get out (or an ambulance could get in) if this baby decided it was time to make his arrival. And this mama ain't no home-birthin' mama. So I sat on the couch with my legs crossed while my husband began to shovel the street. THE STREET.

Finally, we breathed a sigh of relief as we heard the plow arrive. We would be okay.

But then we watched the weather forecast and heard that ANOTHER EQUALLY DETRIMENTAL STORM was heading our way.

Oh, crap.

It was February 24, and I was due February 28. We could not risk getting snowed in again. So I called my doctor, who encouraged me to come to the hospital for an induction. "This way if you're stuck, at least you'll be stuck inside the hospital," she said.

Was I ready to no longer be carrying a nine pound sack of potatoes on my already weakened bladder? Was I ready for a very tall glass of wine next to a giant plate of sushi? You're damn right I was. But I hesitated. "No," I said. "It's too soon. I haven't even reached my due date yet."

After both my husband and doctor assured me that it was safe, the baby was ready, had fully cooked, and I wasn't doing him any harm in inducing labor three days before my due date, I finally agreed. I mean, I reeeeeeally did NOT want to push this kid out in my living room.

But the truth is, I don't think it was about my due date. I knew in my rational mind that this was the best, safest choice and that three days didn't mean anything. I wasn't ready for other reasons.

I wasn't ready to share my baby with the world. I wasn't ready for it to no longer be just him and me. I wasn't ready to say goodbye to this chapter in my life. I wasn't ready to be done with pregnancies.

But I was about to be because this baby was going to be our last baby.

My husband and I had decided, for a myriad of reasons, that three beautiful, healthy children were enough beautiful, healthy children. We'd known from the moment we found out that this baby, girl or boy, was the completion of our family. So, for nine months, I'd tried to prepare myself for this moment.

At the moment of his birth, I would have to accept that this was it. Never again would I have that miraculous experience of meeting a human I'd created. Never again would I see two pink lines, pick a name, and share with my family the news. Never again would I feel a foot or fist kick the walls of my uterus, a home to each of my kids where we first got to know each other. Where for months, it was just the two of us, awake at three a.m., having a talk, wondering what he or she would look like, sound like. What color eyes he would have, or if she'd have Mommy's hair or Daddy's nose.

I was sad that our time was over. As I received the induction medication and began contractions soon after, I tried to ready myself for the inevitable— for saying goodbye to the days of pregnancies. I wanted to stop time as I labored that day, yet I eagerly looked forward to meeting my new son. And that evening, after just a quick push or two, he was here.

And for a brief moment, I was sad. But only for a moment.

The truth is, I knew that it was time to be done. It was the right decision, as our family is complete and whole and perfect. Five is a good number. Five means we can fit in one car and squeeze into one booth at restaurants. We are a little loud, our grocery bill is staggering at times, and my husband and I are outnumbered, but on Friday nights, we all find a way to fit on the same couch for family movie night and pass the bowl of popcorn around.

That baby, born between two blizzards, just turned five years old. He's everything I imagined and has helped my heart to heal. Although I was mourning the end of one of the best chapters of my life, when I held him in my arms and felt his chubby little finger grab ahold of mine, the sadness began to wash away. And as I stared out the window at the snow falling, I knew, at that moment, that everything was exactly as it was meant to be.

VAGINAL BIRTH: ADVICE FROM AUNT PATTI THE GREAT.

JULIE BURTON

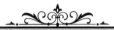

> *"Don't ask the nurses if you pooped on the*
> *table during delivery. They lie."*
> *- Julie Burton, Writer*

She loves you like a mother.
She keeps secrets like a sister.
She hugs you like a friend.

It isn't a riddle. It's an inspirational quote I found on Pinterest. The answer - she is your aunt.

Aunt Becky showed D.J. Tanner how to wear makeup. Dorothy Gale ditched her new friends in Oz to come home to Auntie Em. Julia Roberts played charades with Emma Roberts, thus, fine-tuning the art of acting in her niece.

I lied.

I don't know if Julia Roberts played charades and fine-tuned the acting skills of Emma Roberts. But I would hope Pretty Woman gave her niece a little bit of advice.

My aunt Patti gives me advice all the time.

"You keep pushing that baby out like you're taking a giant shit." - My aunt, Patti.

I met Patti on November 27, 1981.

They say newborns can only see about eight to fifteen inches in front of them. It's just enough for a newborn to see the face of the person holding them. I assume my aunt Patti held me closer than eight inches. As any good aunt would do, she probably held me cheek-to-cheek so I could take in her scent, hear her voice, and feel her skin on my cheeks. She wasn't just my dad's little sister anymore. She earned aunt status.

8,930 days later, my aunt Patti pushed pregnant-me in a wheelchair into the same hospital we met. We were days away from meeting my daughter and Patti's newest great-niece, Emma.

At thirty-five weeks pregnant, my obstetrician ordered me to be on bedrest for high blood pressure. I was told to arrive at every doctor's appointment in a wheelchair. It was too dangerous for me to walk on my own. I don't remember why Patti took me to my doctor's appointment that day. I can only assume my husband, Scott, was at work. I must have asked for availability and Patti came running to my rescue.

I waddled to the front desk of the medical building where Patti asked for a wheelchair to take me up three flights to my doctor's office. A wheelchair was brought out, and I sat. I directed Patti where to go. Patti talked to me from behind as she pushed me down the corridor to the elevator.

Me: "Thanks for taking me, Patti. I don't feel any different when I walk. I could have taken myself."

Patti: "No, you need to listen to your doctor. I'm happy to take you to your doctor today. You know, I'm going to tell you something about labor that no one has probably told you."

Me: "Oh, I've read all the books. Is it the pain? I know. Worst pain in my life. The ten out of ten."

Patti: "The pain is bad, yes, but it isn't about the pain."

Me: "Oh."

Patti: "It's how you know when you need to push."

Me: "The labor and delivery nurse at the class I took said the pain lessens once you're at a ten and your body knows to push."

Patti: "That's true. Did they say what pushing feels like?"

Me: "No, not really."

My wheelchair stopped in the hallway. Patti walked in front of me, and she stared at me.

Patti: "IT FEELS LIKE YOU HAVE TO TAKE A GIANT SHIT, I SWEAR TO GOD. SWEAR TO GOD."

Patti put her arms up in submission.

Me: "Shhhhh! Wait, what?"

Patti: "No one told me this, and I wish they did when I was pregnant. You are my niece, and I will be the one to tell you this. You will feel like you have to poop and you will tell the nurse you have to go to the bathroom, BUT THAT'S THE BABY. It pushes on the same nerves or something. I don't know. Delivering a baby feels like you're taking the world's biggest shit with your legs spread apart in front of everyone. You keep pushing that baby like you're taking a giant shit. Don't worry what others think. Push like you're pooping. It's not poop. It's the baby."

Me: "Oh. Hmm, ok. I'll remember that."

Patti walked to the back of my wheelchair and pushed me through the doctor's office doors.

During the early morning hours of May 24, 2006, Scott and I were in the delivery room. The contractions were intensifying. The contractions turned body-numbing intense, and I couldn't stand to be touched, talked to, or breathed on. I whispered for my family to get out of the room. I wanted to roll in a ball and die.

I later realized my epidural started too late and I felt everything.

Scott rubbed my arm as I felt a contraction bear down.

Me: "Don't."

Scott: "You can do this."

Me: "Just. Don't touch me."

The contraction lifted.

Me: "Ok, ok. I don't like to be touched during those contractions. It's a little better. Oh no. Scott. Scott, I have to go to the bathroom. I have to poop."

Scott: "Ok, I'll call the nurse back."

Me: "No, don't."

Scott pushed the nurse's button.

Scott: "Hey, Julie needs to use the restroom. Can I get some help in here? Thank you."

Patti's voice echoed in my mind – *"Delivering a baby feels like you're taking the world's biggest shit in front of everyone. You will tell the nurse you need to go to the bathroom. That's the baby."*

The nurse walked into my room.

Nurse: "Hey Julie! I know you said you need to go to the bathroom but I'm going to check you really quick."

Me: "Um, ok. I kind of got to go though."

"It's the baby."

Nurse: "Wow, hon! You're at a ten. You flew through those contractions! Your daughter gave you a fast labor. Good job, baby girl! And baby's head is right here! I'll call the doctor. You're ready to push!"

Me: "Scott, I have to go to the bathroom."

Scott: "Can she go to the bathroom?"

Nurse: "No. She needs to stay here. It's common for women to feel like they need to use the bathroom when the baby is pressing down. Your wife's labor went fast. That's good."

Me: "Scott, I'm going to poop all over."

"That's the baby. Push through it."

A medical team filled in the room. Stirrups appeared. Lights from the ceiling hummed down towards my lower torso. The intense pain disappeared. Scott took a leg, and a nurse took another leg. It felt like my legs were being pulled up and off my body, all while feeling the urge to take a giant shit. Every nerve in my body was telling me I had to poop. My legs shook.

"You need to push through it. Don't worry what other's think. Push like you're pooping."

I pushed like I was taking the world's giant shit.

I delivered Emma Burton on May 24th, 2006 at 12:05 in the afternoon. The nurses were impressed with the quick labor, but they were even more impressed with the quick delivery for a first time mom. Emma's quick entrance into the world came from the help of the words from her great-aunt Patti.

Patti visited her newest great-niece later that day.

As any good aunt would do, my aunt Patti held Emma cheek-to-cheek. Emma took in her great-aunt Patti's scent. She heard Patti's voice. And she felt Patti's skin on her cheeks.

My aunt Patti wasn't just an aunt anymore. She earned great aunt status.

LIFESTYLES OF A WOMAN IN LABOR...
C-SECTION WISHES AND PERCOCET DREAMS

DANIELLE SILVERSTEIN

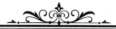

> *"Remember that everyone's experience with*
> *pregnancy is unique."*
> *-Where the Eff is My Handbook*

When I was pregnant with my first child, so many people told me to avoid having a C-section at all costs. I spent nine months praying to the labor goddesses to spare me from the dreaded procedure. At the same time though, something told me that it would be just my luck that somehow, I would wind up having one.

I started having strong contractions two days before my scheduled delivery date. It was around five thirty in the morning and my husband and I headed to the hospital. I was nervous. But having gained over fifty pounds and experiencing a pregnancy ridden with complications, I was ready to get this kid out. I didn't know how to be a parent, but I knew I was ready to repossess my body as my own. I wanted to eat the rawest, most dangerous sushi that Anthony Bourdain's No Reservations could feature. I wanted to make up for the nine months I had spent avoiding drinking wine at restaurants because it just wasn't worth the sideways glances I would receive. I wanted to do all the questionable things I do to my body without feeling the guilt of having another human being growing inside of me (Who am I, even, to be delegated that responsibility?).

The next ten hours were a nightmare. The doctors were sure that I was not in labor and I should go home. I fought with the doctors and nurses for what felt like forever. It turned out I was in labor that entire time, I just seemed to be the only one who knew it. I missed the window for the Epidural. I pushed and pushed, and there was no progress. I always knew

I would be the person who actually couldn't push something the size of a watermelon out something the size of a lemon. I was right. I looked around and hated everyone.

Never had I felt so alone and misunderstood. No one, in the history of the world, had ever felt so much pain. This is what it must feel like to be water-boarded, whipped, punched in the face, and have my ankles broken simultaneously. Only this had to be worse. I started begging for a C-section. Finally, the angels appeared and rolled a wheelchair into the room. The nurses danced me away to what would be the closest to heaven I would ever get. I was sure that all my dead relatives would be there in the operating room waiting for me, singing Hallelujah as I entered through the gates.

They hoisted me up onto the table. I saw the needle the size of a sword from The Princess Bride, and all I could think of was, "stick me, Inigo Montoya, I am prepared." I had to sign a document warning that I could die, be paralyzed, or have a stroke, but it all felt like a small sacrifice to the healing gods.

The needle went in and I truly, in that moment, felt such incredible bliss and euphoria. I lost all feeling from the neck down, and the doctors proceeded to take out my insides in order to finally lasso and capture the little person who had been wreaking havoc in there for so long. There you are you little pain. I love you so much. Now someone, please bring me a bottle of wine with a long straw. No? Too soon? Damn.

I honestly don't know why so many people told me not to have a C-section. During my pregnancy, it was almost as if people would talk about a C-section as "failing"…like if I had to have one it would be a second class delivery or something. I completely disagree. I left the operating room and asked the nurses if it was too early to schedule the procedure for the rest of my unborn children. "No, I don't know when they'll be born, but just block out most of 2008 and 2011 for me, thanks."

They rolled me into my room, and I was told the best news ever. I would get to stay in the hospital for four whole days! For those of you who struggle with math the way I do, that's three extra days of free childcare whenever I wanted it, Percocet, and experts teaching my husband and me how to dress, bathe, feed, and swaddle a newborn. Three extra days to steal all kinds of supplies that we had not yet bought for this child whose parents were clueless about how the hell to have a baby. Ok, so I had to wear a diaper, and I'll forever have a large smiley-face-shaped scar across my lower stomach, but mostly, I was beyond happy with the way things had turned out. I wanted to go to all those people who had made me so fearful and say "why did you do that? Everyone's experience is different, and there is no reason any of us should feel like less of a woman for whatever ensues in our labor and delivery."

I had two more pregnancies, and with both, I felt a relief in knowing what my future held as far as delivery. I looked forward to hospital sleepaway camp when I would sleep whenever I wanted, and everyone was so nice to me. I'm actually sort of bummed I'm not having more kids. Not because I want them, but just because I often dream about that TV remote that never gets lost because it's attached to the bed, and that button I can press and people just bring me stuff. So don't fear when you find out you're going to have a C-section. It's not worth it. Any situation we're dealt is a good one, as long as we come out healthy, and with a happy baby. We're all just trying to get through it all the best way we know how.

PREGNANCY IS UNPREDICTABLE

DINA DREW DUVA

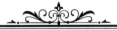

> *"Yes, you are the boss! Too bad 'everything' in your life –including your baby bump- wasn't listening."*
> ~ Mom Cave TV

When I found out I was pregnant with my first child in 2005, I read every pregnancy book I could find. I'm not great with "not knowing," and research is one of my things. If I don't know something. I seek out the answer. After doing my normal due diligence, I KNEW I wanted the epidural. I know that I'm not great with pain. My friends who already had children all said, "Make sure to get the drugs," and according to my research, it was safe.

It was one day before my due date, and I was having weird spotting and pain, so my doctor recommended I have some tests done. Unfortunately for me, the baby heart monitor test was happening at the local hospital, and while I was there, I went in to actual labor. I was bleeding, and the beginning contractions were starting. I was basically at the hospital "too early" which anyone who's had a baby at the hospital will tell you is a BAD idea. My doctor gave me Pitocin to speed things up, and my gosh, the pain was terrible.

I had read about Pitocin but reading about it will not do the pain it causes justice. It's like running a marathon without ever running a fifty-yard dash. It gives your body NO time to adjust to the contractions. So, in came the anesthesiologist with the epidural. Once the drugs kicked in I felt better, but that's when the real party started. My heart rate started to go all over the place, and my daughter's heartrate REALLY started to fluctuate. I was pretty calm during most of this, but everyone around me was beginning to panic, my mom, my aunt, my husband.

Never in all my reading did I come across the passage where it said that you could be allergic to the drugs in the epidural, yet according to the delivery room nurses, it's rather common. (Maybe they should be the ones writing pregnancy advice literature.) A few hours later, I hit around eight centimeters, and my doctor pulled the plug on the epidural and told me that I had to have a C-section. Apparently, there had been talk between my doctor and my family about this already, and perhaps I overheard, but I was really in a state of shock at this point.

I thought I KNEW so much, yet NONE of this was going as I THOUGHT it would.

The drugs began to wear off, and then the pain came back, it was excruciating. I was about to be wheeled in for the C-section when another pregnant woman who was under my doctor's care came in and needed to push. So, I had to wait. I thought being in a smaller hospital would make my birth more intimate and less likely for crazy intervention. Once again, I THOUGHT wrong.

By the time the doctor was ready for me, I had dilated completely. I asked if I could push, but he said it wasn't safe. I felt cheated. Here I had gone through all the work to get to the point where you could push the baby out, and now I had to have the C-section anyway!

The drugs at this point had completely worn off, and now I had to wait another fifteen minutes for the surgery anesthesia to kick in. So, there I was lying on a surgery table, feeling the tug and pull of the procedure, and I was in shock. How did this happen? This wasn't something I had planned.

The recovery after a C-section isn't a ton of fun. It's a painful three or four weeks, letting your abdominal muscles heal. Coupled with the adjustment of a new person to take care of and breastfeeding and no sleep. It wasn't something I was prepared for.

We did survive though, and four years later I was pregnant again. For the third time. The one in the middle of all of this I lost. At seven weeks. My mother had just died from breast cancer, and on the day of her viewing I found out I was pregnant with number two. I lost it at seven weeks. I said that already didn't I? Seven weeks. I felt silly mourning a pregnancy that was over before it even started, but I did. I cried so hard. At the loss of my mom, at the loss of whomever that would have been. No one talks about miscarriages much. Thus, by default, I think I chose to bury it in that place in my heart that I rarely travel to.

My husband and I waited till it was safe to try again, and three months later we were pregnant for the third time with my second child.

From the start, my doctor had recommended I have a C-section. He was "old-school

"and the thinking was once a C always a C. I didn't want a C. I didn't want another surgery, didn't want to go through that crazy recovery, and part of me really wanted to experience what birth was like. I went along though. Even with all my research about V-Bac's (Vaginal after Cesarean), I was too chicken to switch doctors and tempt fate with my body. I mean come on, I was allergic to the drugs in the epidural. I didn't want to chance fate again with going against my doctor.

It was one month prior to my due date, and I was set to go to the doctor, time to schedule the C. I woke up feeling paranoid. All the sudden I was worried I didn't have a bag packed for the hospital. Which was illogical because I had a month to go before my scheduled C. What was a packed bag going to do for me? I packed it anyway. What I didn't know, but was about to find out, was that I was going to experience what it was like to really labor. Perhaps my mom was listening to my silent wish.

I was having cramps all morning, and at about eleven I went to see my doctor. I told him how was feeling, and he checked me, and said, "You are nowhere near ready to have the baby. I am scheduling your C for one month from now. It's Braxton Hicks. Go home." He said it with such conviction, and his words wormed through my head for the rest of the day.

I picked up my daughter from pre-school, went home to give us lunch, and then felt such a panic that I didn't have the right color cover for my nursing pillow. In my need "to know" things, I of course knew I was having a boy, and the pink pillow cover just wouldn't do. I needed a proper cover and I needed it NOW! I dragged my daughter to Sears, and now I'm having more pains. Just like the worst cramps ever, but I keep hearing my doctor's voice in my head. "It's Braxton Hicks, go home." So, I pushed it off.

Lucky for me, my daughter had a playdate scheduled for that afternoon. I drove my daughter over to my friend's house, told my friend how I was feeling, and she told me to go home and lie down for a while. So, I did. I remember laying there in my bed, praying to my mom in heaven. "Mom please help me, how can get I through the next month, if these pains are Braxton Hicks?"

Now remember, I never fully labored with my first. I had had the Pitocin. So, I didn't know what real early labor felt like.

As I lay there I began to count the times between my cramps, and they were consistent. About ten minutes apart. Around seven-ish I went to go get my daughter from my friend's house. As I was waiting at a traffic light, a REAL contraction hit! A whopper! I made it to my friend's house and she took one look at me and told me to sit down on her couch.

She wouldn't let me leave, thank god. At this point I was now having major contractions. They couldn't be real labor pains; my doctor had said so. I sat at my friend's house for the next hour and proceeded to breathe through my "Braxton hicks." My friend finally insisted that we go to the hospital. I argued, but my doctor told me I wasn't in labor, I have a C- scheduled in a month. Well she said, the worst they could do is send you home. My friend brought me home to get the bag I had packed, and maybe I wasn't so crazy after all. Maybe I "knew" something.

By the time we got to the hospital, I was six centimeters and fully effaced. So much for Braxton Hicks. The young but wise residents attending to me at the much larger state of the art hospital which I had so wisely picked for this second pregnancy, asked me if I wanted to try a VBAC. They said I was a perfect candidate. It had been five years since my C-section, which was a good amount of time for my abdominal muscles to heal.

I didn't hesitate. "Let's do it," I said. My slightly shocked friend asked, "Don't you want to wait for your husband." And I immediately responded with a calm and conviction I never really knew I had. "It's my body. It's my decision." It was what I wanted all along and I had such faith in the residents. I told them about the reaction to the drugs in the epidural the first time, and they were on it. They said they had something they could give me in the line for that. My husband rushed to the hospital from his job in New York City. A few hours and three pushes later, my son was born.

He was perfect and didn't even have to spend any time in the NICU. He saved me another month of pregnancy and ten extra pounds.

And here's the funny thing about this whole second go around – the pain I had had with real labor was NOTHING compared to what I endured with the Pitocin. Also, it was so wonderful to wake up the next day and not go through what I went through with the C-section. I felt GREAT the next morning, and not having to heal from a major surgery, made the first few weeks with my new son so enjoyable.

Who knew?

That's the thing about pregnancy, and motherhood for that matter. You can read up on it all you want, but until you live it, you'll never know for sure exactly how it will go.

MY THIRTY MINUTE EMERGENCY AT HOME LABOR

GAIL HOFFER-LOIBL

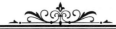

*"Move as much as you are physically (and medically) able.
Even a short walk can lift your spirits and
ease the discomfort of pregnancy."*
~ Maybe I'll Shower Today

"The baby's coming!" I screamed, beckoning my husband to come to the bedroom.

"Close your legs," that's what my husband said, "Close your legs." As if a baby barreling down my birth canal could be stopped by merely squeezing my legs together. Sorry, hun, no amount of Kegels was slowing this baby down.

He caught on quick, and once my husband realized I wasn't going anywhere, he grabbed some old towels (I try not to think about how clean they were) and called 911. With one hand holding his smartphone and the other down by nether region, my husband delivered our baby with guidance from the dispatcher.

Our second baby boy was now in my arms.

I have nothing against home births. I think they are beautiful, and I know for many they are a transcendent experience. Perhaps if the circumstance arose, I would consider one for myself. I would take the proper precautions to ensure my baby was delivered safely with minimal risk to the child and myself.

I never planned to have my second child at home, yet there I was, lying on our bed with little warning he was on his way.

But, before I can talk about his birth, you need to know about how his brother was born.

My first pregnancy was uneventful. Uneventful is as about as perfect a word you can get for a pregnancy. There were no scary trips to the emergency room or demands of bed rest. I commuted to my New York City job, I exercised regularly and walked everywhere. Yes, I experienced morning sickness and the typical aches and pains of carrying a child, but nothing that was enough to cause concern.

While I was experiencing my normal, low-risk pregnancy, I was dutifully following the lessons of my Lamaze class, heeding the advice of my doctor and reading every chapter of my pregnancy books. I was gearing up for what I expected to be a long, difficult labor, and bracing myself for the possibility of medical intervention.

At my thirty-seven week appointment, my doctor examined me as usual, and there was, thankfully, nothing to be alarmed about. I asked her if I might go into labor soon. She said, not likely, as my cervix was barely dilated. Like most first pregnancies, this one was probably going past Thirty-nine weeks.

My body had other plans, because later that week, in the early hours of a Friday morning in November, I woke up with my pajamas slightly wet, thinking I had one of those late pregnancy bladder accidents. And my cervical plug is gone. I woke my husband up to let him know I was in labor and to get ready to ride out the next few hours with me before we had to go to the hospital.

"Come in when the pain gets bad," was what my doctor advised when we discussed when I should go to the hospital once I was in labor. She reminded me how often women come in only to be turned away for not being dilated enough.

Those words reverberated in my head an hour later, as my contractions grew more intense. I toughed out the pain, convinced I was only at the start of my labor journey. I was determined not to go into early, lest I be saddled with a bunch of tests and drugs and sidetrack my plans for natural labor. My fear of medical intervention kept me from truly hearing what my body was trying to tell me.

Well, I couldn't ignore my body for long, as I soon found myself dizzy, nauseated and on the verge of passing out. I was also losing a lot of blood. Baby or no baby, I couldn't stay home any longer. My pain was subsiding, but my anxiety grew.

As my husband relayed my symptoms to my doctor, I lay on the couch, trying to make sense of the sudden urge to push I was now feeling. Feeling immobile, I needed my husband to dress me and help to the elevator. I freaked out, convinced the baby was making its way out of my body. My husband calmly assured me that wasn't the case. He was wrong, but like me, he was not expecting this baby to come so quickly.

Because even when I am in the throes of active labor, I still want to be considerate, I had enough sense to grab a towel in case the baby decided to come out in the taxi. Fortunately, traffic and a skilled driver were on our side, and we made it to the hospital without incident. The cabby missed out on a cool story but left with clean seats.

November 2012 was not a great time to have a baby. Our hospital happened to be one of the few still operating fully after Hurricane Sandy, which meant fewer resources available to the abnormally large number of patients. Getting a wheelchair involved my husband making some strong demands, and the staff no doubt thinking I was a woman overreacting.

Wheelchair obtained, I was brought to a little room where the doctor on call would examine my cervix to see how far along I was. I guess the procedure would then involve me going to one of the labor and delivery rooms to await the arrival of my doctor and deliver the baby.

Instead, the doctor on call took one look between my legs and announced I was crowning. With my husband barely making it into the room, I pushed for less than a minute and was greeted by the cries of a beautiful baby boy. All told, my first labor and delivery clocked in at a little more than three hours.

An hour later, my mom arrived, joking how she even took her time to get to the hospital because how long first labors usually take. Next came my doctor, who immediately suggested I think about scheduling an induction for my next child. I was too physically, mentally and emotionally drained to think about any of that. I had a healthy baby, and a healthy me.

Two years later, I was pregnant for the second time. Armed with my experience from my first pregnancy, I was determined to make it to the hospital on time. I would be hyper-aware of the signs of labor. I would listen to my body.

I chose not to be induced because I still wanted to avoid medical interventions, and I truly believed I knew my body well enough to handle another fast labor. Under the care of a midwife this time, I had the support I needed for natural, in-hospital labor.

How then, did I end up with the entire fire department in my bedroom staring at me holding a newborn?

Every birth story is different, and you can't rely on your past experiences to get you through labor. With my first, I failed to realize the pee "accident" I had was my water breaking, had I known; I would have made it to the hospital much sooner, as this is what most medical providers advise you to do, to avoid infection. However, this time my water didn't break until the moment I felt the urge to push. I was this close to having an en-caul birth, or a baby delivered in the amniotic sac, and probably would have if I was in the hospital.

If my water didn't break, surely the contractions would have clued me into the impending arrival of my baby. Except, there were no contractions. And my mucus plug? No changes there, either.

I was blissfully unaware for the entire day before I went into labor. I even went for a walk and had Mexican food, which I realize now is what you do when you want to speed things up, not slow things down.

Around two a.m. the next morning, I was awakened by a horrible stomach ache. I felt awful and thought maybe I was struck with a bout of food poisoning or perhaps a bad bug. I knew going to the hospital was probably the right call given my condition, but first I wanted to rest for a bit and regain my composure.

As I lay down on the bed, I felt compelled to reach my hands down my pants. My fingers landed between my legs and touched what I knew was a baby's head.

My second baby took about thirty minutes to be born, without warning and once again shattering my birth plan. His speedy and unconventional arrival lead to some significant scares for his survival. Miraculously, under the care of an excellent medical team, he pulled through and is now a thriving soon-to-be three-year-old.

I spent a long time feeling guilty about not doing more to ensure a safer delivery. I wondered if choosing not to induce was the right decision. But, as my midwife reminded me, most providers won't induce before thirty-nine weeks, and my second son came at thirty-eight. So, even if I had made plans to induce, I would have ended up in the same place, perhaps more upset because I had prepared for something much different.

After two lightning fast and unconventional labors, I have accepted that I will be a high-risk patient should I ever decide to have a child again. This reality makes me wonder if I could ever be comfortable putting myself and a baby through the dangers of another fast delivery.

My birth stories are unusual – under two percent of deliveries qualify as precipitous labor, or labor occurring around three hours or less. I say this to calm any fears and assuage any worries. However, I never expected to be one of the two percent, and I listened to what conventional wisdom told me, instead of heeding the guidance of my own body.

Pregnancy books, your doctor, your friends, those hours of Lamaze class – all of those things are fabulous resources and should guide you on your path to delivery. But, don't forget about your greatest resource, your instincts. If something feels off, don't ignore it, even if it means going to the hospital and being sent home.

And, if you happen to notice your labor speeding up, maybe skip the Mexican food.

Beyond Pregnancy

BREASTFEEDING: FIVE THINGS YOUR LACTATION CONSULTANT FAILED TO MENTION

ASHFORD EVANS

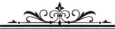

> *"The only advice I have for you is to stop listening to everyone's advice. You'll figure it out."*
> ~ Biscuits and Crazy

1: It Hurts

She may have even gone so far as to tell you "It doesn't hurt." This is a lie. If at first the latch doesn't kill you then you have the wonderful feeling of contractions every time your baby hooks up, and we all remember how good those feel. Once you learn to get through this pain by breathing deeply for the first 30 seconds, you will most likely get cracked, sore, and/or bleeding nipples. When this begins to heal is about the time your milk comes in. Holy hell. Your boobs turn into giant hot swollen throbbing bowling balls. Enjoy. This is just the first week.

Then things begin to mellow out a bit. You think to yourself "Gosh I'm glad I got through all of that. This breastfeeding thing isn't so bad after all." This is when your baby begins teething. Does he want the eighteen dollar Sophie the Giraffe that you bought him? No. Does he want the gel teethers that you keep in the fridge for him? No. He wants your nipple. He wants to clamp down and chew and maul your nipple. Finally, the teeth break through, and you think "Thank God! Some relief!" No, ma'am. He now has teeth. Get ready for this. Every time he chomps down you scream and jerk him off your nipple. Then he cries because you scared him. Congratulations. You're a jerk. You scared your baby. Go ahead and feel that mom guilt.

Finally, he will learn not to bite down after this happens enough, but now he is curious about the world around him. This will cause him to latch and unlatch one thousand times every minute. If you're lucky, he will also begin to grab, knead, pinch, and squeeze your nipple. This my friends is about the time you start googling "Weaning."

2: Strange People Will See Your Nipples

It's not enough that as your lactation consultant was introducing herself to you, she was grabbing your boob and massaging your nipple. You can stomach this indignity. I mean you just had your hoo-ha on display for upwards of ten people you don't even know. Be prepared for anyone and everyone to see your nipples. It could be your husband's eighteen-year-old employee that stumbles upon your car during a pumping session. (He still cannot make eye contact with me without blushing.) It could be the sixteen-year-old girl who walks in on you in the rest stop restroom as you are hooked up right there on the counter because the only outlet in the whole place is in between the sink and the paper towels. (Think of this as a Public Service Announcement warning against teen pregnancy.) It could even be the airport security guard who just keyed into the "family restroom." (There are no words for this one.) But it will be someone somewhere. Just be prepared to leave your pride in your underwear drawer next to all your bras that don't come equipped with an easy access panel. You'll get to wear them again I swear.

3: You Will Let Down at Strange and Inappropriate Times

Yes, she told you about letting down when you talk about your baby, hear your baby cry, think about your baby, see your baby, etc. But she neglected to tell you that you will also let down every time you take a shower. Get used to bathing in a mixture of bath wash and breastmilk and hope it is good for your complexion. There are other strange times that you will let down. With baby number three I let down every single time I brushed my teeth. Weirdness. Just invest in an Amazon Subscribe and Save auto shipment of breast pads.

4: You Will Talk About Breastfeeding to EVERYONE

It's like the filter between your brain, and your mouth gets clogged up with all the milk. You will begin discussing breastfeeding with anyone and everyone who makes the mistake of engaging you in a conversation. It starts out innocently enough with your new momma friend's husband. But it quickly spirals out of control. You will lose the ability to distinguish between appropriate and inappropriate people for this discussion. It could be the group of salesmen at the boat show your husband is participating in. It could be your realtor that you ran into at the grocery store. The cab driver who questions why you need dry ice and what you are shipping (breast milk home from a business trip). Your boss (hopefully a man) when you have to explain why you "need to take a quick break." I have found that hotel concierges are particularly squeamish- it's even kind of fun to watch them squirm as you discuss your "perishable items" that require a mini fridge.

5: Your Hormones Are Worse Than When You Were Pregnant

You may be under the impression that your hormones will return to normal a few months after giving birth. Nay nay my friend. Breastfeeding hormones make pregnancy hormones feel like a day at the spa. Say hello to our newest resident of crazy town. An email about an extra dance practice for your five-year-old the same week you are traveling for work? This is enough to send you into a full-on shower crying session that may outlast the hot water in your water heater. (We all do that right?)

You spilled four ounces while trying to make a bottle? This feeling of failure can last for days. Don't worry the dog will lick up the milk. You forgot to put the milk in the fridge, and now it's spoiled? It's cathartic watching your tears swirl together with the sour milk as they spiral down the drain. Oh, and the whole "You won't have your period till you stop breastfeeding"? Another lie. If you are one of the lucky ones, who does get an early return from your monthly visitor just know that because of all the crazy screwy jacked up hormones raging in your body that it won't be normal. I had my period for two months straight. TWO FREAKING MONTHS!!!!

So there you have it. The skinny on what you won't learn about in the free breastfeeding class that you dragged your husband to.

THE BOTCHED EPIDURAL FROM HELL

KRISTEN HEWITT

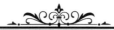

> *"Don't weigh yourself and don't compare yourself to others.*
> *Scales and Instagram are joy-stealers"*
> *- Kristen Hewitt, Writer.*

"So you're not going home, you're having a baby today." My OB announced at my thirty-five-week checkup. In his office my blood pressure was super high from pregnancy-induced hypertension, so he sent me down to the hospital below his office to be monitored.

After the fog of surprise wore off and they wheeled me to my room to give me the Pitocin, I was bold, brazen, and overconfident when I announced to the nurse, "I won't need an epidural...PU-LEASE", complete with an eye roll.

After living with stage four endometriosis, and several surgeries including an ovarian torsion, pain was my middle name. I had cramps since middle school that left me doubled over for days. The grapefruit-sized endometrioma (blood filled cyst) twisted my fallopian tube for nine days before I realized this was something more than my normal horrendous cramps. (Which resulted in the loss of that ovary. Oops!) The injections and blood tests I suffered through for seven years going through insemination and in vitro fertilization had braced me for the worst. My body had been a punching bag for every treatment known to man...a few contractions I could handle.

And I was right - for the first five centimeters.

Contractions were nothing in the early phase of labor. For me, they were just short cramps, not nearly as bad as what I had experienced my whole life. I loved being able to walk around and go to the bathroom 18,000 times. Because that's what contractions felt like to me, horrible back pain and pressure so bad I felt like I had to poop. Like non-stop. Until I got to around five centimeters. Then the pain was starting getting worse, and coming fast. It was nearly 8:00 pm and I wasn't sure if I wanted an epidural, but if I dilated much more they wouldn't be able to administer it. So I gave in.

The anesthesiologist was almost off duty after a twelve-hour shift. When she entered the room, the contractions were coming every five minutes, and I was exhausted. So was she. She wanted my husband to leave the room, but I begged for him to stay. She was not pleased and quite frankly not the kindest person on the planet. She needed me to be still so she could administer the epidural, but see the problem was when a contraction came I would quake with pain. My husband tried to hold and brace me, but it felt like a tornado of action. She would bark and scare me. I would jump and shake during a contraction, and that's when it happened.

I felt the burn of the epidural like an awful bee sting and immediately screamed, "OH MY HEAD!"

The pain was unlike anything I had ever experienced, and they knew what had happened. She had to re-do the epidural again, and I sobbed with fright. I was told I had a spinal headache. Basically, when a needle enters your spine, there is a chance that the needle can nick or puncture the Dural membrane of the spine. This causes spinal fluid to leak and leads to what's known as a spinal headache. After an epidural during childbirth, this only happens one or two percent of the time. Lucky me, I was in that two percent.

When you have a spinal headache, it's not just a headache. It's the most excruciating pain you will ever feel if you try to lift your head off the pillow. If you are horizontal, then the fluid doesn't leak. But when you stand up, the angle of your spine causes the fluid to leave, and you immediately feel such extensive pressure and pain that you literally can't move. Can't walk, can't eat, you have to remain flat on your back.

I immediately felt this directly after my hellish epidural procedure and during childbirth. Once our miracle baby came just after 10:00 pm I was given a choice, have a blood patch, a procedure where they do yet another epidural and fill the hole in your spinal column with blood from your arm. Or drink mass quantities of caffeine.

I did the Dew. Mountain Dew that is. I couldn't bear a third epidural of the day. Caffeine and bedrest sometimes did the trick, so I followed their orders. And two days later I was a little better and was released from the hospital, leaving my premature baby in the NICU.

But when I got home, the headaches came back and worsened. I couldn't get out of bed, eat, shower, or go to the hospital and visit our sweet miracle baby. The one we had prayed for – for seven years. The one I desperately wanted to hold and nurse. But instead I laid alone in my bed, my womb empty, my heart shattered, and my head pounding. I pumped milk every two hours for my mom and husband to take to Lila, our daughter, while I cried silently waiting for someone to return. For someone to help me to finally feel better.

After two days of agony, I knew I needed to get some help. We went in through the emergency room and were given a private room. A new anesthesiologist came and did a battery of tests. Because lying flat didn't immediately resolve my headache, he wasn't sure that a blood patch was the answer. He thought I could be feeling a stress or a tension headache. They gave me the option of the blood patch, but I wrongly refused.

Back at home, it took me another few days of agony to realize I did, in fact, need the blood patch…and fast. I had to go back through the same emergency room, this time, though it wasn't cushy. I had to lay on the hospital room floor to get relief. Then later they moved me to a gurney in the hallway. And after waiting fourteen hours for the anesthesiologist, still pumping milk every two hours, I finally received the patch at 3:00 AM. Five days after her birth and five days since holding my baby.

The time apart from her was heart-wrenching. I had felt her kick and hiccup for eight months in my belly, and then poof, she was just gone.

I couldn't see her. Couldn't hold her. Couldn't touch her little fingers. Couldn't comfort her.

Would she even recognize me?

The time between the blood patch and my husband wheeling me to the NICU felt like slow motion. But even in the middle of the night, the room was illuminated by the buzz of the overhead fluorescent lights, and I went to her. Finally off the lung machine now wrapped in a BiliBlanket (for jaundice) they handed Lila to me.

And I nursed my baby.

There's absolutely no way to describe the relief I felt in that moment. How my uterus contracted with the touch of her mouth to my nipple. How I wept knowing that she and I would finally be OK. And how right it felt to hold her in my arms. It was a like a piece of my heart I never knew was missing, finally was there.

We may not have had an easy start, but I learned so much from my botched epidural experience from hell. To be my own patient advocate. To listen to my body and trust in my own intuition and inner voice. And to never have an epidural again from an anesthesiologist who was almost off duty.

And yes, even after this traumatic birth experience, we did do IVF once more. It miraculously worked and resulted in our second daughter. And when it came time to deliver early once again, you can bet I asked for the head of the anesthesia department to administer my epidural first thing in the morning.

And it worked like a charm.

JOY RECLAIMED - HOW POSTPARTUM DEPRESSION REFINED ME, BUT DIDN'T DEFINE ME

LAUREN EBERSPACHER

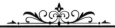

"My simple pregnancy advice is…this too shall pass."
-From Blacktop to Dirt Road

"Oh, my word. Isn't he just the cutest thing ever?" she exclaimed as she came up and stroked my baby boy's cheeks. There is something about a baby that attracts every old woman in church, isn't there?

"He is, isn't he?" I forced a smile and bounced my son in my arms. "He's just the best baby ever."

He is a good baby, I thought to myself. I don't know why I don't feel as happy about it as I should.

"And how about the big sisters, do they just love him, too?" she asked.

"Oh my goodness, they can't get enough of him! They love him so much," I replied.

I wish I loved him that much, too. Why can't I feel anything for this baby? I know what I'm supposed to feel for him, I know how this is supposed to be. What is happening to me?

It was just a few weeks prior to this interaction at church that I had started to feel myself slowly slipping away. Our house had been hit hard by the cold and flu season, I hadn't slept in weeks, and I was overwhelmed, overworked, and underappreciated.

But there was something else. I had started to feel less joy. It was getting harder to find it in the everyday mundane – playing on the floor with my girls, cuddling with my baby at bedtime, dressing up my newborn, going out for dinner on a date. These were all things that used to bring me joy. But for some reason, I couldn't muster anything up. Not only that, but I wasn't interested in them at all.

But I thought I could push through. That if I could fake it long enough, I might come out of the fog and no one would notice. So I posted cute baby pictures on Instagram and Facebook, I flashed the biggest smiles I could when I was out of the house, and I did everything I could to hide what I was feeling from those closest to me. Especially my husband. And all the while, I slipped farther and farther away.

Until one day I woke up completely lost.

You have to get up. You can't stay here forever; I tried to convince myself.

It was a few weeks since the conversation with the old woman at church, and things had gone from bad to worse.

I could hear the baby crying in the pack-n-play out in my bedroom. My girls were out in the living room watching cartoons. They had been there for two hours.

You have to go and get the baby, I said to myself. He needs you. The girls need you, too.

That was just it. I was so needed. Needed by three little people and a grown man and all of them needed something different every hour of every day. There were meals to make, dishes to scrub, laundry to wash, crafts to clean up, diapers to change, spit up to wipe away, baths to give, stories to read, noses to wipe, hugs to be given, and a marriage bed that had been cold for far too long. I was so needed, and my cup was so empty.

But I didn't want to fill it back up again.

I had no desire to do anything but lay there on my closet floor.

There was also something new that started this week. A scream.

A silent scream in my head that I somehow had to get out. A scream that haunted my moments of loneliness came rushing in when another thing was added to my day and an eerie voice that consumed my mind. It crushed me.

And so there I was on the closet floor. Sobbing. Screaming. Crying out for someone to take away the darkness that shrouded my mind and had held my heart captive.

But that was just the thing. My heart had always been held captive with joy. A joy that was encompassing. Consuming. And holy.

I heard the garage door open, and my husband pulled his truck into the garage. It took everything in me to get up off the floor and stop crying, but I managed to get up off the closet floor and pick up my baby before he came in the door.

I wasn't sure how much longer I could go on without telling him.

I became a Christian as a little girl. I was five years old when I decided to walk with Jesus, and from that point on I experienced the joy that only he could bring. I do not remember a time without having God be a part of my life; therefore I do not remember a time without joy. That was why the absence of joy was so confusing to me.

I thought that something like this wasn't supposed to happen to me. I loved God, and I was the daughter of the King! So why was the joy of the Lord that I had always experienced not coming through and being my strength and saving me from this darkness? Was I not praying hard enough? Was I not trusting? Was I not strong enough in my faith?

These questions swirled around in my mind every day. It became exhausting trying to mask my problems, ask these questions, and try to fix my soul on my own. I knew I needed help. I knew I needed to reach out. And I knew that I had to start with him.

He had been distant for weeks, and he didn't even know how to talk to me anymore. Leaving for work during the day and working out in the garage on his truck at night. I knew that I had become unbearable to live with, and I knew he was struggling to understand where his wife had gone to. But to tell him how broken I was and to let him see me in the shame of my darkness? It was almost too much to bear. But I knew that it had to happen. It was just a matter of when.

We were sitting in our living room, he was on one couch, and I was on the other. He was browsing on his phone, and I finally got the courage to tell him what I was feeling. "Um, honey I think we need to talk. I think I have postpartum depression. Like, I know I'm different. I think I have a problem."

Without looking up from his phone, he replied, "Well if it's that bad why don't you go to the doctor and get some medicine or something." That was it. I lost it.

"That's not what I need you to say!" I screamed at him. "I need you to come over here and put your arms around me and tell me you love me and that I'm going to be OK. I'm not OK!" My screams turned into sobs, and he walked over across the room. For the first time in months, he looked at me. And he saw me.

"Oh, honey... Honey, I had no idea. I'm so sorry. I know now, I'm here."

And that conversation changed everything. He saw. He understood. And from there on out, I had his support, 100%. But we never would have gotten to that point if we I hadn't been brave enough to tell him what was wrong. If I hadn't had the courage to take on step out of the darkness and back into the light.

I sat on the edge of the table at the doctor's office, the crinkly paper beneath me. This was one of the hardest, most shameful days of my life. But it was also one of the most necessary and important. By involving my doctor in my postpartum depression, it gave me valuable insight from someone who had experience and knowledge. It also gave me the opportunity to start on antidepressants. And the day I filled my prescription, I took my little white pill, and I never looked back.

Not because the person in the mirror isn't enough. But because I want to be the best version of who God made me.

Not because I believe that God can't heal my mind if He chooses. But because I believe He gave people the wisdom to make this medicine to help people like me.

And I took my Little White Pill because I love my husband. I wanted to be a wife who could stand by my man and give him what he needed like he stood by my side and supported me in my moment of need.

And I took my Little White Pill, not because I was a bad mom, but because I wanted to be a mom who could love her kids fully. Because I wanted to be giggling and playing with them on the living room floor more than I was curled up and crying on the closet floor.

Not because I want to be the person I used to be. But because my mind and my heart are being made new. Postpartum Depression is and always will be a part of my story. And I've come to realize that that's ok. It has changed me. I will never be the same.

But it does not define me. And today, I've reclaimed my joy, and I am no longer lost. And I'm walking back in the light.

WHAT I WISH I KNEW WHEN I WAS PREGNANT ABOUT BECOMING A MOTHER

MIA CARELLA

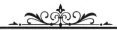

> *"During this pregnancy and throughout your journey into motherhood, you will learn so much, experience so much, and feel so much. No matter what, please remember that you are never alone. Not ever."*
> *~ Mia Carella, Writer*

Dear Former Self,

Congratulations, mama-to-be! I see you reading those two little pink lines. Pretty surreal, isn't it? Crazy and exciting at the same time. As the seconds on the timer ticked by, I know how your anticipation grew and how much you were hoping to see that positive result. This is something for which you have hoped and prayed for so long.

Oh mama, there is so much I need to tell you! So much that you don't know right now about the journey you are about to embark on. Through pregnancy, childbirth and motherhood you will learn so much. I know you think you are prepared. You have read pretty much everything you could get your hands on about pregnancy and becoming a mom. After all, it's been all you have been thinking about for so long. But, I need to tell you that what they say is true. No matter how prepared you think you are for all of this, you really cannot be ready for what is to come.

Here are some things that you need to know:

1. You know that your body will change as you grow this baby, but you don't really know. Your breasts will get huge, and then later deflate like tired party balloons. Your belly will stretch larger than

you thought would be physically possible. (Oh, and it doesn't go back to normal the minute the baby arrives. Plan to be in maternity pants for weeks – ok, months - afterwards.) And, your ability to control your bladder will diminish after your body is put through the ringer. Yes, it's all true.

2. You don't know that shit happens. Literally. Yes, you have heard the stories about what can happen on the delivery table as you push out your beautiful, new bundle with everything you have. These stories are also true. I repeat, this is not a drill! But, don't sweat it. The nurses and doctors won't bat an eyelash, and in the chaos of it all your husband won't notice (or if he did he was kind enough to never speak of it again).

3. You don't know that once you become a mother you will appreciate little things that you always took for granted. Things like shirts without spit up stains and the sound of a vacuum cleaner. (Who knew a vacuum could lull a cranky infant to sleep? Answer: Apparently everyone with a baby.)

4. You don't know that you will do things you never thought you would do after having a baby. Gross things. Weird things. Like sucking boogers out of your baby's nose with your mouth. (Yes, this is a thing. They even sell equipment for it.) Also, eating partially chewed food off your child's plate. Disgusting, right? Not anymore. A mom's got to do what a mom's got to do.

5. You don't know that although you will be gaining a beautiful baby at the end of the next nine ten months, you will lose a lot of things. For example:

Your sense of modesty. See #3 above. Once you poop in front of others, modesty pretty much goes out the window.

Sleep. Oh, so much sleep will be lost! Stock up on those naps while you still can. Seriously. Please. I'm begging you.

Some hair. Do not panic. It is entirely normal to shed a little after baby is born. Do not be alarmed when looking at the bathtub floor after your showers.

Personal space. There will be another little person with you (if not physically attached to you) for the majority of your life from now on. Although the circumstances may change over the years of motherhood, this mere fact of having a perpetual human shadow will not. Please don't squander the uninterrupted toilet time you have now. You will miss it when it's gone.

6. Speaking of losing things, you don't know that you will actually feel like you are losing yourself for a little while. This is something no one warned you about. You will go from being a woman, a wife, a friend - an individual - with your own hopes and goals, to fading into the background as your newborn takes center stage. Your sole purpose will become "giver and sustainer of life" and your own agenda will disappear. In fact, sometimes you will wonder if maybe you disappeared. It may seem at times that you are invisible. Don't be afraid. This won't last forever. I know it feels that way, and the tunnel may seem long and dark, but you will find the light and yourself again as you learn how to incorporate your new role as mom into your life.

7. You don't know that sometimes things don't go as you had hoped. Sometimes things will happen that weren't in your master plan. Maybe a test result during pregnancy that you didn't expect to receive or news that you didn't expect to hear. Different does not necessarily mean bad. It means just that – different. It will be ok. You will adapt and you will change to accommodate the variation in your path. You are stronger than you know.

8. You don't know that you are going to need to learn to cut yourself some slack. I know you are used to holding yourself to high standards and getting all the things done. It is going to be challenging to do everything that you are used to doing after the baby comes. The house will not be clean for a long while and

your daily to-do list will seem to never shrink. I know this may be shocking, but you might not even get a shower every day. It's ok, mama. No one expects you to be perfect. Everything will get done. Keep loving your baby and doing the best you can. And most importantly, ask for help if you need it. You have so much support around you. Please take advantage of it.

9. You don't know how many new experiences and new worries you will have. So, so many. You may feel isolated at times and feel like you are in unchartered territory. You will find yourself doing Google searches at all hours of the night and scanning mom group message boards to find out if other people are going through the same things as you. The quick answer is yes. Yes, they are. You are never alone. Never, ever.

10. You cannot possibly know how this new love will change you. Yes, of course you know you will love your baby. Of course, your little one will become your priority in life. But, no, mama. You do not know the intensity of the love you are about to experience. It is the kind of love that will envelope your whole being. The kind that will color your perspective on life in every way. The kind that will make you want to do everything to change the world for this new, little person. No, you will never be the same after this love. Not one little bit.

11. You don't know that this will be the most difficult, but most wonderful job you will ever have. Despite all the sleepless nights, cold cups of coffee and moments of feeling like you are at your wit's end, you will always, always be thankful that you are a mother. Motherhood by design is full of ups and downs. Trust me, it's all worth it.

There is so much you don't know yet, but you will learn. Oh, how you will learn.

I am so excited for you. I know your joy is mixed with some uncertainty right now; wondering if you have got what it takes to do this whole mom life thing.

You will be great, mama. I just know it. Congratulations!

Love,

Me

EATING CHOCOLATE IN THE BATHROOM: TIPS ON MOTHERHOOD

REBECCA HASTINGS

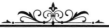

> *"You are going to get some things wrong in this whole parenting journey. You just will. But you are also going to get a lot of things right."*
> *– My Ink Dance*

I stood in the bathroom, back to the door ignoring everything happening on the other side. I unwrapped the small piece of chocolate and tried to take a deep breath. This wasn't in my plan. In fact, most of this wasn't in my plan.

Motherhood was supposed to be beautiful, and sweet baby smells and chubby toddler cheeks asleep at night. No one told me there would be a day that hiding in my bathroom eating a piece of chocolate to escape for two minutes would be my reality. Sure, people had tried to tell me, but that wasn't going to be me. Those parents were exaggerating, telling their mom version of "I caught a fish this big" stories.

I hid in the bathroom eating chocolate in the middle of the day.

I asked for an extra project at work just for a few more minutes of quiet.

I was up thirteen times last night.

Exaggerations.

Right?

And then I became a mom. Those "big fish" stories were feeling less like stories and more like a horror movie. They weren't all bad. There were good things like loving so intensely it brings you to tears or the pride you feel when you watch your little one accomplish something new.

As many expectant moms do, I had my fancy pregnancy book prominently on my nightstand, like a Bible. I had dog-eared pages, underlined vital things, and spilled food on it trying to balance a baby belly, a book, and a snack.

But eventually, the baby comes. And while you still turn to that book, you realize a little more every day that this parenting job has no manual. There are some things no book can prepare you for.

To help you out I've compiled a partial list. In no particular order because parenting seldom has order (that gem is just a bonus).

1. Sleep will never be the same. You will sleep through the night again. Probably. But it's different.

   A friend told me that he never understood. People told him he would be tired. He is a firefighter. He jumps up at all hours to save the day. But he said he had no idea what tired was until he had his baby.

2. The love you feel will be more profound than you can imagine. But it may not happen instantly. Give yourself time to grow into your new role with your new little one.

   Giving you and your baby time to grow into new things is going to be required more than you know. This is a good place to start.

3. You will never be ready for your child's first steps. You think you will. You may even grab the video in time. But those first steps are the beginning of their ability to walk to amazing things, and not all of them will be you.

4. Ditto their first date. I mean, how can we really be ready for this? But knowing that none of us are and we all survive creates a solidarity of sorts.

5. There is seldom a clear right answer. Growing up they taught us that there was right and wrong. Period. No in between. As a parent you see that there is usually just a choice between two things, neither one completely right or wrong. And that's okay.

6. The things that you think should come naturally sometimes don't. It's okay to say it's hard and seek help (and it's okay to change course.) In fact, modeling this for our kids is a wonderful gift.

7. "The Talk" is not one and done. And you will have to have "the talk." Talk once and keep talking. Little talks, small conversations. The more we talk about the uncomfortable things the more likely our kids will be to come to us when they need us most.

8. Leaving them home alone for the first time is hard. And it's still hard the 100th time. There will be a day when these people that you arrange whole schedule systems around are capable of being home alone. You will leave every number you know in case they need it even though you will be back before they can dial. It's harder for you than it is for them. It will become more natural.

9. They will get hurt. The hurt that is better with a Band-Aid is the easy kind. There are heart hurts that are much harder, and you will want desperately to fix it. But they don't need you to fix it as much as they need you to be there with them through it.

10. Your presence is more important than having all the answers. Be there in the middle of whatever they are going through. But remember that it is okay to hide in your bathroom with a chocolate bar when you need a break.

11. We all feel like we are failing as parents at some point. It probably means you're great enough to care. Keep going.

12. Having a baby changes your relationships. All of them. It's not necessarily a bad thing. You'll develop an intimacy over this shared person with your spouse. Your mom friends will understand you

in a way others have not. And your friends without kids will be a fun escape when you need it.

13. There is so much joy. Be on the lookout because it can be like shooting stars. You can miss it if you're not looking. Always look for joy. Even in the ordinary.

14. Sleep deprivation is far more than being tired. It can bring all the feelings…overwhelmed, cranky, and unable to concentrate. But you will get through it. Find what works for you because it is important.

15. That milestone you're stressing over (When will she walk? Why isn't my baby talking? Will she ever learn to tie her own shoes?) will come. As my pediatrician told me, they won't go to college in diapers. Relax a little.

16. Cluster feeding is a real thing. And it's exhausting. But it is temporary.

17. Having baby #2 or 3 or 7 is different from the previous ones. You have more to juggle. Give yourself (and your babies) some grace. And yes, you will be able to love them all. Love is funny like that; the more you love, the more you seem to have.

18. It won't be like this forever. Kids are always changing. Remember that in the hard places.

19. Post-partum depression is real. And it may not look the way you thought. Be aware of you as much as you are aware of your baby. There's no shame in it, it's nothing you did wrong, and there is help.

20. It is not always about you. Your little one has feelings and ideas and will make decisions all on their own. Not everything they do is a reflection of you as a parent.

21. No book has all the answers. **THE END.**

ABOUT THE AUTHORS

Jennifer Bairos lives in Toronto, Ontario, Canada with her husband and her son. When she's not blogging, Jenn teaches middle school, reads avidly, exercises sometimes, and drinks caramel macchiatos. Her writing has been featured on Mental Health on The Mighty and in *The Unofficial Guide to Surviving to Life with Boys*. Find more from Jenn on her blog <u>www.asplendidmessylife.com</u> as well as on Facebook @asplendidmessylife and Instagram @jennbairos.

Mary Ann Blair is a stay-at-home mom living in the Pacific Northwest with her two little gentlemen and hubs. She loves connecting with other parents who like to keep it real! Her work has been published on Her View from Home, Perfection Pending, That's Inappropriate, Pregnant Chicken, and Red Tricycle. She can be found at miraclesinthemess.com or fb/MiraclesInTheMess.

Lyndee Brown is Haden and Ryland's mom. She has been married to her husband Matt for ten years. She has a bachelor's of science degree and works as a Respiratory Therapist during the day. At night she moonlights as Superwoman. She is very fluent in sarcasm and can burn toast with the best of them. She is the co-founder of the blog hashtagllifewithboys.com.

Julie Burton is a wife, mother, writer, and bacon-hater living in Overland Park, Kansas. She is a columnist and contributing writer for *SIMPLY KC magazine*. She contributes to Sammiches and Psych Meds, Mock Mom, The Good Men Project, My Life Suckers, and The Today Show. She is also an ambassador for *National Geographic Kids*. Burton also is an author in the anthology, *But Did You Die? Setting the Parenting Bar Low*. And yes, she really does hate bacon. Please, don't drop her as a friend.

Mia Carella is a stay-at-home mom and writer who lives with her husband and their two children. She likes reading, napping and spending time with her family. She dislikes cooking, cleaning and adulting in general, but absolutely loves being a mom. Her work has been published on Scary

Mommy, Babble, Love What Matters, The Mighty and more. Read more on Mia's website, www.ThisMomWithABlog.com, and follow her on Facebook, Twitter, Instagram and Pinterest.

Aaronica Cole is a once single but now married, homeschooling mom of 3. When she's not battling with her children to do school work or trying to freestyle her way through unschooling, you can find her blogging her way through life at TheCrunchyMommy.com. As if she has spare time, the time she does have is split between helping other businesses develop with strategic marketing campaigns and sewing her family's wardrobes. She's been featured on TheKitchn.com, Huffington Post, Red Tricycle, The Curvy Fashionista and VoyageATL Trailblazers.

Alison Chrun is the mother of two beautiful boys and the author of her blog, Appetite for Honesty. When she's not writing about the brutal truths of her life, she's enjoying all that her cozy bed and trash reality television has to offer.

Dina Drew Duva, mother of two, is a professional actress who has appeared on shows like *Limitless, Law & Order: SVU, Blue Bloods, White Collar* and *Rescue Me*; as well as dozens of television commercials. She is also a writer/blogger/photographer/producer/meme maker and co-owner of MomCaveTV.com. To learn more about her visit www.dinadrew.com.

Lauren Eberspacher is the author and speaker of the blog From Blacktop to Dirt Road where she gives heartfelt Biblical encouragement for the everyday mama and wife. She and her husband Eric live on their grain farm in southeast Nebraska with their three small children. Her devotional, *Midnight Lullabies*, is being released in April of 2019.

Ashford Evans lives with her husband, three children, and three dogs in South Carolina. When she's not pregnant, breastfeeding, or polishing off a bottle of wine she is busy holding down her sales career or working at their family owned business. She blogs about her crazy escapades and living life in between being the bread winner and the bread maker at biscuitsandcrazy.net. Most recently she became known as "the urinal cake lady" (for real ya'll google it). She has been featured in US Weekly,

Independent Review Journal, Pop Sugar, Mom Babble, Scary Mommy, and the Huffington Post.

Joey Fortman is a twenty plus year on-air radio/television vet, turned MOM, took her career to a whole different dimension when she left the full-time radio business in 2008 to bring her story to life online. With real life recovery of Postpartum Depression, Joey started blogging through her loneliness, depression & real life identity crisis. Watching the digital destiny of women fade away because of the behavior of other women online, Joey started Real Mom Media & Reality Moms to give women a real place to be themselves. Reality Moms share stories of motherhood through all walks of life. Joey is a contributor to many digital outlets including Quirky Momma & Kids Activities Blog where she hosts a travel/tech & toy show to over 3.2 million fans. Aside from Reality Moms, Joey has taken her voice to *Good Morning America*, *Today Show*, *Dr. Oz*, *Nick Mom*, *The Talk*, *Dr. Phil*, *Fox & Friends* and so many more. When not laughing with her kids, Joey can be found face first in her *Swear Word Coloring Book*.

Brook Hall has always wanted to make people laugh, lucky for her she gave birth to two hilarious boys who give her more than enough material to work with. She spends all her time at home taking care of her two little comedians, while also trying to squeeze in moments alone with her hubby. Brook can be found on her blog Stay Home Mama. Her favorite times of day are nap time, bed time and when she gets a new "like" on Facebook.

Meagan Haltiwanger Saia is a part-time gifted teacher and a full time mom to her adorable little boy Owen. Meagan believes in the power of sharing our stories and her writing can be found at lifeofowen.wordpress.com.

Rebecca Hastings traded the classroom for writing when she stayed home with her three children. Passionate about authenticity, faith, and family, she now writes regularly at www.myinkdance.com. She has also been featured on multiple sites including The Washington Post, For Every Mom, The Mighty, and Money Saving Mom. Her first book, *Worthy*, is available on Amazon. A wife and mother of three in Connecticut, she writes imperfect and finds faith along the way.

Abigail Hawk is an award-winning New York-based actress who has worked on television shows *Body of Proof, The Jim Gaffigan Show, The Beautiful Life*, and *Are We There Yet?* Most recently, she guest-starred opposite Mariska Hargitay and Raul Esparza on *Law and Order: SVU*. But perhaps she is most recognizable as feisty Detective Abigail Baker, the unflappable right hand of surly but lovable Commissioner Frank Reagan (Tom Selleck) on CBS' *Blue Bloods*. Hawk's silver screen work includes *Almost Paris*, which was directed by Domenica Cameron-Scorsese and premiered at the 2016 Tribeca Film Festival. She also starred in the creative indie feature *Bubble Girl*, due for release late 2018, served up some sassy salon owner sauce in rom-com *Rich Boy, Rich Girl*, and played opposite Chevy Chase and Howard Hesseman in the feel-good holiday feature *A Christmas in Vermont*. Abigail currently resides on Long Island with her husband, two sons, dog, two cats, four fish, and one snail. Her favorite foods are chicken salad and cannoli and her favorite color is green. The fastest way to her heart is through coffee, wine, and following her on Instagram.

Karsson Hevia is an Author, *The Unofficial Guide to Surviving Life with Boys*, mother to two little dudes, and a content writer, blogger, and social media strategist working in the Bay Area (while maintaining her deep Midwest roots.) Karsson writes about the excruciatingly beautiful juxtaposition of motherhood and her continual desire to find the so-called balance of life on her blog: 2manyopentabs.

Gail Hoffer-Loibl is the mom of two loud, spirited, loveable boys who are endless source of inspiration for her writing. Her blog, Maybe I'll Shower Today, captures the raw, beautiful and often humorous aspects of motherhood and raising two young men. Her work has been featured on Her View from Home, Scary Mommy, That's Inappropriate and more. You can follow her on Facebook and Instagram @MaybeIllShowerToday and on Twitter @BloggerGail.

Whitney Hsu is wife to Ryan, and mom to three awesome kiddos under 6 who daily toe the line between hilarious and offensive. She's the mama behind the blog We're Only Hsuman, and her writing has been featured on Everyday Exiles, Perfection Pending, Mom Babble, and Scary Mommy.

She "retired" from teaching music to stay home with the kids, then picked up two other jobs writing and leading worship at her home church in North Carolina. When she's got a rare moment to herself, she's gardening, running, or reading.

Bianca Jamotte LeRoux is a mom, award-winning filmmaker, actress, writer, and creator of the series *Real Mommy Confessions*. Her acting career began in musical theater and quickly turned to commercials, print, and recurring roles in soap operas *One Life to Live* and *As the World Turns*. Bianca's first venture into moving behind the camera was the short film *Twinkle*, directed by Rosalyn Coleman. *Twinkle* was the Brooklyn Girl Film Festival winner for Audience Choice in 2014. Bianca was the co-writer, co-producer, and star of the film. *Real Mommy Confessions* has won numerous awards, and most recently Bianca was honored with the Alice Guy-Blache Women in Cinema Award from the Golden Door International Film Festival for her work as the writer, director, producer, and star of the dramatic short *Flush the John*.

Karen Johnson is a free-lance writer and mother of three who loves beer, wine, and bacon and lives with her family in the Midwest. She works as assistant editor at Sammiches and Psych Meds and is a staff writer at Babble, Scary Mommy, and Her View from Home. You can follow Karen on Facebook, Instagram, and Twitter as The 21st Century SAHM.

Dana Kamp is the founder and content creator of 39ish Life, as well as a freelance editor and writer. Her writing has appeared on Today Parents, The Huffington Post, Perfection Pending, Sunshine and Hurricanes, That's Inappropriate, Parenting Teens and Tweens, and in the book *The Unofficial Guide to Surviving Life with Boys*. She is currently working on a children's book series and a book chronicling her journey as a surrogate. She lives in Florida with her hot husband and their four amazing boys. You can follow along with their crazy, fun, emotional, loud life on Instagram and Facebook @39ishlife.

Britt LeBoeuf Hailing from the Adirondack Mountains of Upstate New York, Britt has a background in Human Services and Child Development. Britt is a married mom to a loving husband and two beautiful boys. You can find her first self-published novel, *Promises of Pineford* on Amazon and Lulu. You can also find her at These Boys of Mine by Britt LeBoeuf and on Facebook. Her work can also be found on Scary Mommy, Her View from Home, That's Inappropriate, Blunt MOMS, Today Parents, and Organized Mom.

Karen Galinsky Lesh is a tap-dancing, poetry-writing, chocolate-loving, fulltime working mom of THREE BOYS (who are pure rascal with a side of sweetness). She thrives on creative expression through rhythm and rhyme, and connecting with others through stories. When she's not cleaning a toilet (3 boys!!!), breaking up a wrestling match, enjoying family time, or working her corporate job as a Marketing Director, she blogs about the adventures of being a Mother of Boys (M.O.B.) at M.O.B. Truths (www.mobtruths.com). Her work has been published on Scary Mommy, and Karen is excited to keep sharing her parenting tips/tricks, relatable stories and lots of laughs through her blog.

Kristen Hewitt is a two-time Emmy Award Winning Reporter and Host for *Fox Sports SUN* and the Miami HEAT, writes a parenting and lifestyle blog at Kristenhewitt.me, and hosts a podcast *Be Who You Want to Be*. Her work can also be seen and covered on *US Weekly, Pop Sugar, The Today Show, The Huffington Post, A Plus, She Knows, Scary Mommy*, to name a few, or you can follow her on Facebook, Instagram, and Twitter. Kristen's favorite job though is raising her two daughters. She tries to teach them to live every day with grace, gratitude, love...and a lot of laughs!

Holly Loftin is a wild child, turned wife and mom, who is just trying to get by one long day at a time. She writes for the blog **From the Bottom of My Purse**, where she shares her humorous and real stories about her life as an underachieving mom. She's opinionated, sarcastic, and most of the time, over-caffeinated. You can find her over at Scary Mommy, Huff Post Parents, and many places in between. For more, follow her on **Facebook** and **Instagram**.

Andrea Mullenmeister is a freelance writer based in Minnesota. She is a mother to her warrior son who was born more than four months before his due date. Andrea writes about her family's story of love, hope, and survival at www.AnEarlyStartBlog.com. Her essays about motherhood, prematurity, and parenting a child with extra needs have been featured nationally. She loves to grow good food, play in the woods, and laugh with her family.

Tiffany O'Connor is the author, freelance writer, and blogger behind #lifewithboys. She is the co-author/editor of *The Unofficial Guide to Surviving Life with Boys*. Her work appears in several anthologies, including *Chicken Soup for the Soul My (Kind of) America*. She has written for several media outlets. Tiffany is a mom to two amazing, energetic, and fearless human boys and one loveable furry boy dog. She is married to her high school sweetheart and has three college degrees. Her hobbies include watching television shows about zombies, hiding in her hot tub with a glass of champagne, and listening to Taylor Swift songs on repeat.

Sunayna Pal was born and raised in Mumbai, India, Sunayna Pal moved to the US after her marriage. A double postgraduate from XLRI and Annamalai University, she worked in the corporate world for five odd years before opting out to embark on her heart's pursuits - Raising funds for NGOs by selling quilled art and became a certified handwriting analyst. Now, a new mother, she devotes all her free time to writing and Heartfulness. Dozens of her articles and poems have been published and she is a proud contributor of many international anthologies. Her name has recently appeared in *Subterranean Blue Poetry, Cecile's Writers* and *Poetry Super Highway*. She is part of an anthology that is about to break the Guinness world of records. Know more on sunaynapal.com

Michelle Price is the founder of Honest & Truly! (https://honestandtruly.com) where she shares engaging solutions for our modern busy lifestyle. She took her years of experience in management consulting, marketing, and account management and turned it into a creative outlet that has taken off. Her love of food lets her share the recipes her family (read: recipe testers) enjoy so others can recreate them, as well as her other obsessions of travel and technology. She's found the joy in combining stories and solutions that drive readers to her site and also allow her to partner successfully with brands who see the benefit of storytelling in campaigns. She lives in Chicago with her husband and two children where she's always on the lookout for more food to share on Instagram (@honestandtruly).

Holly Rust is a native Texan but currently resides in the great city of Chicago with her husband and two sons. She's a writer, author and global entrepreneur helping women be their best self. She is the creator and voice behind A Mother's Guide to Sanity, a lifestyle blog where she shares stories about raising two rambunctious boys all while trying to manage her life and career. Her work can be found in several anthologies available on Amazon. You can also find her on Scary Mommy, Huffington Post, *Good Housekeeping* and *TODAY.*

Louise Sharp is a mum of three. She started off blogging around six years ago, mainly to deal with her daughter's journey with autism and her diagnosis process. She saw blogging as a way of expressing her thoughts and feelings. From that she began training as a Journalist, but her passion for writing always lays with writing about issues close to her. Issues others could possibly relate to. She started to blog about living with and beating depression and anxiety, being an advocate of ending the stigma surrounding mental health issues. She's had articles in a variety of publications, including Thrive Global and in the local press. She now blogs for a living, writing about anything from days out with her family, to product or service reviews to provide content for local businesses and services

Danielle Silverstein is a SAHM of three kids and two rescue dogs. Her blog, Where the Eff Is My Handbook, is meant to help moms out through support and humor. Check out her podcast, *Marriage and Martinis*, coming soon! You can follow her on Facebook and IG.

Rachel Sobel is a South Florida native (via Long Island like the rest of em). Living the NEW normal: Marriage, Baby, Divorce, Remarriage, another baby. In between navigating massive loads of laundry, cooking thirty-two different meals for picky eaters, doing ponytails over until they are perfect with "NO BUMPS, MOM!" and double fisting iced coffee, she finds time to blog all about it at Whine and Cheez-its. Her work can be found on Pop Sugar, Scary Mommy, the Huffington Post and she also hosts a podcast about motherhood called *The Keep It Real Moms*. While she's pretty Type A, she admits that you are more likely to find baby wipes and a half-eaten bag of Cheez-its in her purse than cash.

Karen Szabo is a part-time worker by day, boy-mom by night, and blogger at www.theantsybutterfly.com any time in between. She's doing her best to keep her sanity by writing about life as an anxious mom. She's a contributor for The Mighty and has written for some of her favorite sites such as Mom Cave TV, Sunshine Spoils Milk, Sammiches & Psych Meds, Perfection Pending, and Scary Mommy. Karen can be found on Twitter @AntsyButterfly, Instagram, and Facebook where she shares her truths about surviving this wild parenting world.

Briton Underwood is a proud father of three boys. You can find his words published both online and in print under the moniker Punk Rock Papa. When not raising children or writing, he works on being a trophy husband for his beautiful wife.

Stacey Waltzer hit her forties running complete with a teaching career, husband, and two little kids. Not realizing that life could get even more chaotic, she started to write and hasn't stopped since. With real life stories that read like fiction, she exists with the help of caffeine and lots of laughter. Her writing has been featured on various blogging sites and she is excited to be making her way into the world of published writing. If you would like to contact her, always search under the pile of laundry first.

Amy Weatherly loves red lipstick, graphic tees, and Diet Dr. Pepper a little more than she probably should. Most days you can find her lounging in sweatpants, running kids from one place to the other like a crazy person. Her family is her home and her passion is helping women find courage, confidence, and the deep-rooted knowledge that their life has a deep and significant purpose.

LETTER FROM THE EDITOR

Thank you for reading this book. We hope you enjoyed it. This is our second anthology. If you have a son, are pregnant with a son, or just want to understand what it's like to raise boys you should read our first book, 'The Unofficial Guide to Surviving Life with Boys.' You will love it.

When we started this journey, I was expecting it to be easier than the first time around. Just like I expected my second pregnancy to be easier. I was wrong both times. The past few months were filled with ups and downs. I can't even begin to express the gratitude I feel towards are contributors. I hope that each one of the writers and the artist who contributed to this book knows just how much I appreciate them for standing by us during all of the struggles and missed deadlines that happened due to circumstances beyond our control. If you loved their stories (or Heather's cover art) as much as I do make sure you check out their books, blogs, Facebook pages, Twitter feeds, and fabulous Instagram posts.

This book was created with the goal of sharing what it is really like to be pregnant. Every pregnancy is different, unique, and special in its own way. I am hoping that you are able to relate to at least one (hopefully more) of these stories and that some of the advice that was shared helps you during your pregnancy journey.

Please tell all your pregnant friends about this book…or even better make it your new go-to baby shower gift. If the baby keeps you up late and you need something to do we would love for you to write us a review on Amazon.

Congratulations on your pregnancy!!!

XOXO

Tiffany

#Lifewithboys